Quick & Easy
DIABETIC RECIPES

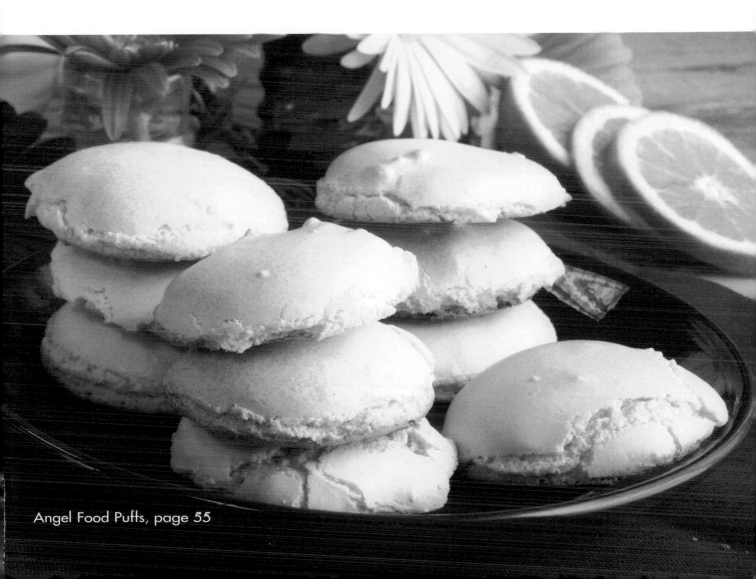

Angel Food Puffs, page 55

Turkey Pepperoni Pizza, page 134

DELICIOUS WAYS TO CONTROL DIABETES

Quick & Easy
DIABETIC RECIPES

Compiled and edited by
Anne C. Cain, M.S., M.P. H., R.D.

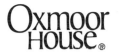

Oxmoor
House®

Library of Congress Catalog Number: 2002-141306
ISBN: 0-8487-2516-6
ISSN: 1523-8032
Printed in the United States of America
First Printing 2002

Be sure to check with your health-care provider before making any changes in your diet.

Editor-in-Chief: Nancy Fitzpatrick Wyatt
Executive Editor: Katherine M. Eakin
Art Director: Cynthia R. Cooper

Delicious Ways to Control Diabetes
Quick & Easy Diabetic Recipes

Editor: Anne Chappell Cain, M.S., M.P.H., R.D.
Copy Editor: L. Amanda Owens
Editorial Assistant: Diane Rose
Director, Test Kitchens: Elizabeth Tyler Luckett
Assistant Director, Test Kitchens: Julie Christopher
Recipe Editor: Gayle Hays Sadler
Test Kitchens Staff: Jennifer Cofield; Gretchen Feldtman, R.D.;
　　David Gallent; Ana Kelly; Jan A. Smith
Senior Photographer: Jim Bathie
Photographer: Brit Huckabay
Senior Photo Stylist: Kay E. Clarke
Director, Production and Distribution: Phillip Lee
Books Production Manager: Theresa L. Beste
Production Assistant: Faye Porter Bonner

Contributors:
Designer: Carol O. Loria
Indexer: Mary Ann Laurens
Photo Stylists: Melanie Clarke, Connie Formby
Medical Advisor: David DeAtkine, Jr., M.D.

Cover: Banana Split Cake, page 54

Contents

Dear Friends,

As a person with diabetes, sometimes it seems that all I do is think about when to eat, what to eat, or how much I should or shouldn't eat! And as a busy person, it's often a challenge to make sure that I take time to stay on my meal schedule and eat appropriately.

But even though diabetes demands that you take time to eat, it doesn't demand that you spend a lot of time cooking. With *Quick & Easy Diabetic Recipes,* you can get good-for-you food on the table in minutes. Our staff of registered dietitians and cooking experts have put together over 130 easy recipes, all with no more than 30 minutes of work time. **SuperQuick** recipes and **make-ahead** recipes are flagged for easy reference. Plus, we give you a **one-week menu plan** with a whole week of 20-minute meals! The ingredient lists are short, and the methods are simple.

> # One of the very nicest things about life is the way we must regularly stop whatever it is we are doing and devote our attention to eating.
>
> **LUCIANO PAVAROTTI and WILLIAM WRIGHT**
> *Pavarotti, My Own Story*

Each recipe has nutrient information and exchanges, so you can easily work the food into your meal plan. You'll also get must-have diabetes nutrition information and the steps you can take today to get your diabetes under control. And for your convenience, we've added "Food in the Fast Lane," a guide to eating out.

Quick & Easy Diabetic Recipes lets you spend time at the table with your family and friends instead of in the kitchen. I guarantee it will be better for your blood sugars as well as your soul.

Sincerely,

Anne Cain

Anne Cain, Editor

nutrition action

Here's the latest in diabetes nutrition information, plus actions you can take today to control diabetes.

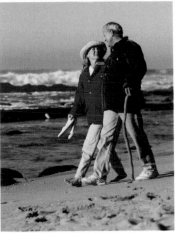

Walk On

Research shows that people who are at risk for Type 2 diabetes can reduce their risk of developing diabetes by 58% by losing as little as 5 to 10 pounds and walking three times a week. For people with Type 2 diabetes, weight loss and moderate exercise can reduce the need for diabetes medications and improve blood sugar control.

Action: Start a walking program today. Begin slowly if necessary, and work up to at least 30 minutes, three times a week.

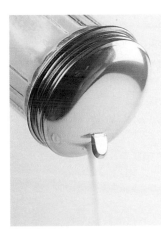

Understand Sugar

The "rules" for sugar and diabetes have changed, according to recommendations from the American Diabetes Association. It used to be that people with diabetes were told to stay away from anything with sugar. But research shows that sugar, when eaten with a meal, does not raise blood glucose any more than a starchy food with an equal amount of carbohydrate.

Action: Pay attention to the total amount of carbohydrate in your diet, including all types of sugar. If you do eat sugar, do so in moderation, and always account for the amount of carbohydrate the sugar provides.

Count Carbs

Carbohydrate counting is a flexible method of diabetic meal planning in which you allot a certain amount of carbohydrate for each meal and snack. Then you decide what you want to eat based on the amount of carbohydrate you have budgeted. In another method of carb counting, you adjust your insulin based on the amount of carbohydrate that you plan to eat, using a predetermined ratio.

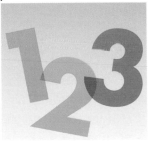

Counting carbs gives you flexibility in eating, but the method requires a good understanding of the carbohydrate content of foods, plus a bit of calculating.

Action: Talk to a registered dietitian or certified diabetes educator about tools and resources for carb counting.

Know Your Numbers

Forget the stock market values and the baseball scores. Here are some target numbers for reducing your risk of heart disease when you have diabetes.

Action: Schedule an appointment for lab work, and ask the doctor to call you with the results. Or go to a health screening. Talk to your doctor about how to improve your numbers.

Test	Desirable Levels
Total Cholesterol	less than 200mg/dl
LDL Cholesterol	less than 130mg/dl
HDL Cholesterol	greater than 45 mg/dl (men) greater than 55 mg/dl (women)
Triglycerides	under 200mg/dl
Blood Pressure	under 130/85

Lose Weight the Right Way

Some aspects of low-carbohydrate, high-protein weight loss plans are appropriate for people with diabetes, especially the advice to limit refined sugars and choose high-fiber starches. However, the rationale behind most of these diets is not based on sound science. Here are some things to remember if you are considering a low-carb diet:

• Carbohydrate is not bad. Sugar is not toxic. If you have diabetes, you must pay attention to the amount and kind of carbohydrate you eat, but the body is designed to run on a proper mix of carbohydrate, protein, and fat. Eating too much of any one of these nutrients can cause weight gain.
• There is no scientific evidence that eating specific types of carbohydrate or eating foods in certain combinations causes insulin resistance and, therefore, weight gain.
• You might lose weight temporarily, but a diet that restricts certain foods and limits choices is usually not effective for long-term weight control.

Action: Consult with your doctor or registered dietitian if you want to try a low-carbohydrate, high-protein weight loss plan.

Fill Up on Fiber

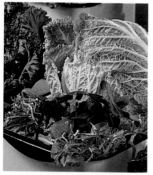

People with Type 2 diabetes can lower blood glucose levels, reduce blood cholesterol, and reduce risk of heart disease if they eat a high-fiber diet. The current recommended amount of fiber is 25 grams per day. But a recent study showed that people who ate at least 50 grams per day were able to lower blood glucose by 10 percent more than the people who ate 25 to 30 grams of fiber. These high-fiber folks also decreased their cholesterol and triglycerides more than people on the lower fiber diet.

Action: Eat more fresh fruits, vegetables, and whole-grain products. Ask a registered dietitian about the best sources of fiber. You can also get fiber information from The American Dietetic Association at www.eatright.org or 800-877-1600.

food in the
fast lane

Use this guide when you just don't have the time or inclination to cook, or when you're traveling. Many restaurants provide specific nutrient information about their menu items; ask the manager what's available. Here are some general tips for low-sugar, low-fat dining in a variety of restaurants.

Salad Bar Finesse

To make the best choices, you should:

■ Walk around the salad bar and look at all the selections before making your choices.

■ Select low-fat items, such as lettuce, spinach, broccoli, carrots, cauliflower, bell peppers, tomatoes, onions, fresh fruit, and low-fat salad dressings.

■ Avoid high-fat items, such as chow mein noodles, pepperoni, cheese, coleslaw, pasta salad, potato salad, bean salad, macaroni salad, pea salad, and regular salad dressings.

■ Select fresh fruit; the canned variety is often in syrup. The gelatin salads are also made with syrup-sweetened fruit.

■ Select broth-based soups instead of cream soups.

■ Count the carbohydrate you get from crackers, croutons, and bread.

■ Eat slowly so that you don't have time to return to the food bar for second helpings.

Learn Chinese

If you are on a low-sodium diet, ask if reduced-sodium soy sauce is available.

■ Leave off deep-fried items, such as tempura, fried won tons and dumplings, egg rolls, crispy noodles, and fried chicken wings.

■ Avoid chow mein items; the vegetables and pieces of meat are fried and served over crisp fried noodles.

■ Avoid high-fat egg foo yong dishes.

■ Request steamed rice instead of fried.

■ Avoid items with "sweet-and-sour" in the title.

■ Pay attention to the portion size of rice. One-half cup of rice has about 22 grams of carbohydrate.

■ Order individual stir-fry items instead of combination plates with fried rice and egg rolls.

■ Ask about the house specialties; some restaurants offer lobster, scallops, or other low-fat seafoods.

■ If you eat your fortune cookie, be aware that 1 cookie has about 5 or 6 grams of carbohydrate.

Master Mexican

The challenge of eating Mexican food is that the menu is very high in carbohydrate, and many items are fried. Use these tips to make healthy choices.

■ Ask the waiter not to bring the basket of chips and salsa, or place it at the opposite end of the table from where you are sitting (12 chips have about 20 grams of carbohydrate and 9 grams of fat).

■ Choose black beans instead of refried beans, which are usually fried in lard.

■ Order items with soft flour tortillas instead of crispy fried corn tortillas.

■ Order an appetizer and a green salad, or order individual items and side dishes instead of the combination plates and platters.

■ Split an order of fajitas. One order is usually enough for two people.

■ Request low-fat sour cream.

■ Ask for the guacamole and sour cream on the side.

■ Use salsa to add flavor instead of high-fat sour cream and guacamole.

■ Leave off the margaritas; they have a lot of sugar.

That's Italian!

Pay attention to the words on the menu when you're ordering Italian foods.

To order reduced-fat Italian dishes, look for these terms:

■ *Al marinara* (with tomato sauce)

■ *Pomodoro* (tomato)

■ *Primavera* (indicates that the dish has vegetables)

■ Lemon-herb sauce

■ Light sauce

■ Lightly sautéed in olive oil

The following terms usually indicate high-fat dishes:

■ Alfredo sauce (Parmesan cream sauce)

■ *Parmigiano* (lightly breaded, fried, and topped with Parmesan cheese)

■ Cream sauce

■ Breaded and fried

■ Sautéed in butter

■ Cheese-stuffed

■ Cheese-filled

Pizza Power

Here are some tips for ordering a healthful meal at a pizza restaurant.

■ Order thin-crust pizzas; they have less carbohydrate than thick-crust pizzas.

■ Select only one meat topping, and choose a lean meat like chicken or lean ham.

■ Do not order extra cheese. The cheese is high in fat and sodium.

■ Pay attention to the sweetness of the tomato sauce; most pizza sauce has a little sugar, but some sauces are sweeter than others. Count in a little extra carbohydrate if the sauce tastes sweet.

■ Order breadsticks only when you are having salad for your meal. Breadsticks plus pizza crust or a sandwich adds up to a lot of carbohydrate.

■ If you order a personal pan pizza, split it with someone else. One pizza has about 76 grams of carbohydrate and counts as 5 Starch Exchanges.

■ Fresh vegetable toppings are low in fat and sodium, and add fiber, vitamins, and minerals.

cooking in the diabetic kitchen

Diet is the cornerstone of diabetes management because the food you eat directly affects your blood sugar. Use this section and the recipe chapters for information as well as inspiration for quick and healthy cooking.

Top 10 Healthy Cooking Tools

Quick and easy healthy cooking is no problem when you have the right tools. Here are the top 10 items our food editors say they can't do without.

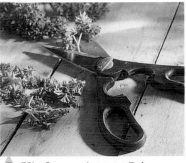

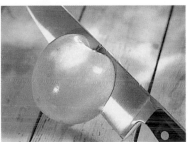

1 Set of sharp knives: Chopping fresh fruits and vegetables is quick and easy when you use sharp knives.

2 Microwave oven: Use for melting, steaming vegetables, toasting nuts, and defrosting, as well as a host of other "quick-fix" steps that will reduce your prep time.

3 Measuring spoons: Select a set of spoons that graduate from ⅛ teaspoon to 1 tablespoon so you don't have to guess at amounts.

4 Dry and liquid measuring cups: Use the appropriate measuring cup, either dry or liquid, so your amounts will be accurate.

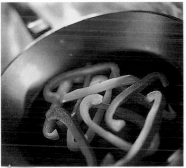

5 Nonstick skillets, saucepans, and baking pans: You don't have to use much fat, if any, when you cook in nonstick utensils. And cleanup is quick and easy, too!

6 Hand mixer: This mixer is great for small, light jobs.

7 Kitchen scissors: Scissors are handy for mincing herbs, chopping tomatoes in the can, trimming fat from meats and poultry—plus many more uses.

8 Instant-read thermometer: A key safety factor is cooking food to the proper temperature, so use an instant-read thermometer to check eggs, meats, and poultry.

9 Steam basket or vegetable steamer: Steaming veggies is a quick and healthy way to cook vegetables because it preserves nutrients as well as flavor.

10 Broiler pan/broiler pan rack: When you broil, much of the fat drips away into the pan, so broiling is a quick and low-fat cooking method.

Stocking Up

Use this handy list to keep your kitchen stocked with the
basic ingredients you need for quick low-fat, low-sugar cooking.

Check the pantry for these staples:
- ☐ Baking powder
- ☐ Baking soda
- ☐ Bouillon granules: chicken, beef, and vegetable
- ☐ Broth, canned: reduced-sodium chicken and beef, vegetable
- ☐ Cornstarch
- ☐ Flour: all-purpose, self-rising, whole wheat
- ☐ Milk: nonfat dry milk powder, fat-free evaporated
- ☐ Oats: quick cooking
- ☐ Oils: olive, sesame, and vegetable
- ☐ Sugar and sugar substitutes
- ☐ Unflavored gelatin and sugar-free gelatin mixes

Keep these fruits and vegetables on hand:
- ☐ Canned beans
- ☐ Canned tomato products: paste, sauce, whole, diced, and seasoned tomatoes
- ☐ Canned vegetables
- ☐ Canned fruits packed in juice
- ☐ Dried fruits

You can always make a meal when you have these grains and pastas:
- ☐ Bulgur
- ☐ Couscous
- ☐ Dry pastas
- ☐ Rice and rice blends
- ☐ Dry cereals without added sugar

Add flavor with these condiments and seasonings:
- ☐ Bottled minced garlic
- ☐ Dried herbs and spices
- ☐ Mayonnaise, low-fat
- ☐ Mustards
- ☐ Salad dressings and vinaigrettes: fat-free and reduced-fat
- ☐ Seasoning sauces: hot sauce, ketchup, low-sodium soy sauce, Worcestershire sauce
- ☐ Vinegars

Fill the fridge with these items:
- ☐ Cheeses, reduced-fat
- ☐ Eggs and egg substitute
- ☐ Milk: fat-free and low-fat buttermilk
- ☐ Margarine, reduced-calorie margarine, and light butter
- ☐ Rolls and pizza dough
- ☐ Sour cream, low-fat
- ☐ Yogurt, low-fat

Stock up, and store these foods in the freezer:
- ☐ Cooked chicken: diced or strips
- ☐ Ground round, pork chops, other meats
- ☐ Frozen fruits
- ☐ Frozen vegetables
- ☐ Juice concentrates

How Much Is a Serving?

For many people, controlling portions is the biggest challenge in controlling diabetes. Whether you are counting carbohydrate or watching portion sizes in order to lose weight, the guide below will help you see in your mind's eye the appropriate serving size for each of a variety of foods.

1 ounce cooked meat, poultry, or fish	=	Matchbook
3 ounces cooked meat, poultry, or fish	=	Deck of playing cards, cassette tape, or the palm of a woman's hand
1 slice cheese	=	3.5-inch computer disk
1 ounce cheese	=	4 dice or a tube of lipstick
2 tablespoons peanut butter	=	Golf ball
1 standard bagel	=	Hockey puck or 6-ounce can of tuna
1 cup potatoes, rice, or pasta	=	Size of a fist or a tennis ball
1 medium potato	=	Computer mouse or 1 small bar of soap
½ cup cooked vegetables	=	6 asparagus spears, 7 to 8 baby carrots or carrot sticks, 1 ear of corn, or 3 spears broccoli
½ cup chopped fresh vegetables	=	3 regular ice cubes
1 cup chopped fresh leafy greens	=	4 lettuce leaves
1 medium orange or apple, or 1 cup fruit or yogurt	=	Baseball

Source: National Center for Nutrition and Dietetics of The American Dietetic Association and its Foundation, ADAF, copyright 1998

menu planner

A Week of 20-Minute Meals

SuperQuick Meals

All of the meals in this plan can be prepared in 20 minutes or less. When you get ready to create some of your own menus, look for the recipes in the book with "SuperQuick" at the top of the page.

Quick and Easy Recipes

The recipes in bold are recipes from this cookbook, and the page numbers are provided for easy reference. The other items—such as fresh fruits, vegetables, breads, and grains—are simple ways to round out the meals.

Calorie Levels

For each day, we've given you three different calorie levels: 1500, 1800, and 2000. The daily calorie percentage is approximately 55 percent calories from carbohydrate, 20 percent from protein, and 25 percent or less from fat. The exchange values for each meal are listed below the menu. Use your own meal plan to determine the specific number of servings you can have or the number of other items you can add.

Personal Meal Plans

Use these menus and the recipes in the book to make your meal plan work for you. Since meal and snack plans differ according to dietary treatments and goals, this weekly menu planner is simply a guide to recipes and food items that make pleasing meals.

MONDAY

	1500 calories	1800 calories	2000 calories
BREAKFAST	English muffin, 1 Low-sugar jelly, 1 tbls Light butter, 1 tbls Scrambled egg, 1 Orange juice, ½ c Fat-free milk, 1 c **2 Starch, 1 Fruit, 1 Meat, 1 Milk, 1 Fat**	English muffin, 1 Low-sugar jelly, 1 tbls Light butter, 1 tbls Scrambled egg, 1 Orange juice, ½ c Fat-free milk, 1 c **2 Starch, 1 Fruit, 1 Meat, 1 Milk, 1 Fat**	English muffin, 1½ Low-sugar jelly, 2 tbls Light butter, 2 tbls Scrambled eggs, 2 Orange juice, ½ c Fat-free milk, 1 c **3 Starch, 1 Fruit, 2 Meat, 1 Milk, 2 Fat**
LUNCH	**Oriental Beef on Rye,** *page 195,* 1 serving **Broccoli-Tomato Salad,** *page 149,* 1 serving Orange, 1 **2½ Starch, 2 Veg, 1 Fruit, 1 Meat**	**Oriental Beef on Rye,** *page 195,* 1 serving **Broccoli-Tomato Salad,** *page 149,* 1 serving Orange, 1 **2½ Starch, 1 Veg, 1 Fruit, 1 Meat**	**Oriental Beef on Rye,** *page 195,* 1 serving **Broccoli-Tomato Salad,** *page 149,* 1 serving Orange, 1 Fat-free milk, 1 c **2½ Starch, 2 Veg, 1 Fruit, 1 Meat, 1 Milk**
DINNER	**Santa Fe Skillet Casserole,** *page 96,* 1 serving Tossed green salad with vinaigrette, 2 c Canned pineapple slices, 2 **1½ Starch, 2 Veg, 1 Fruit, 3 Meat, 2 Fat**	**Santa Fe Skillet Casserole,** *page 96,* 2 servings Tossed green salad with vinaigrette, 2 c Canned pineapple slices, 2 **3 Starch, 2 Veg, 1 Fruit, 6 Meat, 2 Fat**	**Santa Fe Skillet Casserole,** *page 96,* 2 servings Tossed green salad with vinaigrette, 2 c Canned pineapple slices, 2 **3 Starch, 2 Veg, 1 Fruit, 6 Meat, 2 Fat**
SNACK	Graham crackers, 3 Peanut butter, 1 tbls **1 Starch, 1 Meat, 1 Fat**	Graham crackers, 6 Peanut butter, 1 tbls **2 Starch, 1 Meat, 1 Fat**	Graham crackers, 3 Peanut butter, 1 tbls Fat-free milk, 1 c **1 Starch, 1 Meat, 1 Milk, 1 Fat**

Abbreviations Key: **tbls** = tablespoon(s)   **tsp** = teaspoon(s)   **oz** = ounce(s)   **c** = cup(s)   **Veg** = Vegetable Exchange

14

TUESDAY

1500 calories	1800 calories	2000 calories
Frozen waffles, 2	Frozen waffles, 2	Frozen waffles, 3
Sugar-free syrup, 2 tbls	Sugar-free syrup, 2 tbls	Sugar-free syrup, 3 tbls
Sausage, reduced-fat, 1 oz	Sausage, reduced-fat, 1 oz	Sausage, reduced-fat, 2 oz
Blueberries, ½ c	Blueberries, ½ c	Blueberries, ½ c
Fat-free milk, 1 c	Fat-free milk, 1 c	Fat-free milk, 1 c
2 Starch, 1 Fruit, 1 Meat, 1 Milk, 2 Fat	2 Starch, 1 Fruit, 1 Meat, 1 Milk, 2 Fat	3 Starch, 1 Fruit, 2 Meat, 1 Milk, 2 Fat
Beefy Minestrone Soup, *page 186,* 1 serving	**Beefy Minestrone Soup,** *page 186,* 1 serving	**Beefy Minestrone Soup,** *page 186,* 1 serving
Cheddar cheese, 1 oz	Cheddar cheese, 2 oz	Cheddar cheese, 2 oz
Wheat crackers, 5	Wheat crackers, 10	Wheat crackers, 10
Apple, 1	Apple, 1	Apple, 1
	Fat-free milk, 1 c	Fat-free milk, 1 c
2 Starch, 1 Veg, 1 Fruit, 2 Meat, 2 Fat	3 Starch, 1 Veg, 1 Fruit, 3 Meat, 1 Milk, 2 Fat	3 Starch, 1 Veg, 1 Fruit, 3 Meat, 1 Milk, 2 Fat
Steak au Poivre, *page 104,* 1 serving	**Steak au Poivre,** *page 104,* 1 serving	**Steak au Poivre,** *page 104,* 1 serving
Mashed potatoes, ½ c	Mashed potatoes, ½ c	Mashed potatoes, 1 c
Steamed carrots, 1 c	Steamed carrots, ½ c	Steamed carrots, 1 c
Strawberries, ½ c	Roll, 1	Roll, 1
	Light butter, 1 tbls	Light butter, 1 tbls
	Strawberries, ½ c	Strawberries, ½ c
1½ Starch, 2 Veg, 1 Fruit, 3½ Meat, 1 Fat	2½ Starch, 1 Veg, 1 Fruit, 3½ Meat, 2 Fat	3½ Starch, 2 Veg, 1 Fruit, 3½ Meat, 2 Fat
Mocha Smoothies, *page 32,* 1 serving	**Mocha Smoothies,** *page 32,* 1 serving	**Mocha Smoothies,** *page 32,* 1 serving
1 Starch, ½ Milk	1 Starch, ½ Milk	1 Starch, ½ Milk

WEDNESDAY

1500 calories	1800 calories	2000 calories
Whole wheat toast, 2 slices	Whole wheat toast, 2 slices	Whole wheat toast, 2 slices
Light butter, 1 tbls	Light butter, 1 tbls	Light butter, 2 tbls
Poached egg, 1	Poached egg, 1	Oatmeal, ½ c
Orange sections, ½ c	Orange sections, ½ c	Poached eggs, 2
Fat-free milk, 1 c	Fat-free milk, 1 c	Bacon, 1 slice
		Orange sections, 1 c
		Fat-free milk, 1 c
2 Starch, 1 Fruit, 1 Meat, 1 Milk, 1 Fat	2 Starch, 1 Fruit, 1 Meat, 1 Milk, 1 Fat	3 Starch, 1 Fruit, 2 Meat, 1 Milk, 2 Fat
Dilled Chicken Salad Sandwiches, *page 196,* 1 serving	**Dilled Chicken Salad Sandwiches,** *page 196,* 1 serving	**Dilled Chicken Salad Sandwiches,** *page 196,* 1 serving
Carrot sticks, ½ c	Low-fat potato chips, 1 oz	Low-fat potato chips, 1 oz
Grapes, ½ c	Carrot sticks, ½ c	Carrot sticks, 1 c
	Grapes, ½ c	Grapes, ½ c
2 Starch, 1 Veg, 1 Fruit, 3 Meat	3 Starch, 1 Veg, 1 Fruit, 3 Meat, 1 Fat	3 Starch, 2 Veg, 1 Fruit, 3 Meat, 1 Fat
Grilled Tuna with Herbed Mayonnaise, *page 71,* 1 serving	**Grilled Tuna with Herbed Mayonnaise,** *page 71,* 1 serving	**Grilled Tuna with Herbed Mayonnaise,** *page 71,* 1 serving
Greek Salad Bowl, *page 146,* 1 serving	**Greek Salad Bowl,** *page 146,* 1 serving	**Greek Salad Bowl,** *page 146,* 1 serving
French bread, 2 slices	French bread, 2 slices	French bread, 2 slices
Cubed melon, ½ c	Cubed melon, ½ c	Cubed melon, ½ c
		No added sugar ice cream, ½ c
2 Starch, 2 Veg, 1 Fruit, 5 Meat, 1 Fat	3 Starch, 2 Veg, 1 Fruit, 5 Meat, 1 Fat	3 Starch, 2 Veg, 1 Fruit, 5 Meat, 2 Fat
Wheat crackers, 5	Wheat crackers, 10	Wheat crackers, 5
Cheddar cheese, 1 oz	Cheddar cheese, 1 oz	Cheddar cheese, 1 oz
		Fat-free milk, 1 c
1 Starch, 1 Meat, 1 Fat	2 Starch, 1 Meat, 1 Fat	1 Starch, 1 Meat, 1 Milk, 1 Fat

THURSDAY

	1500 calories	1800 calories	2000 calories
BREAKFAST	Bran flakes cereal, 1c Banana, 1 Fat-free milk, 1 c	Bran flakes cereal, 1 c Banana, 1 Fat-free milk, 1 c	Bran flakes cereal, 1 c Whole wheat toast, 1 slice Light butter, 1 tbls Banana, 1 Fat-free milk, 1 c
	2 Starch, 1 Fruit, 1 Milk	2 Starch, 1 Fruit, 1 Milk	3 Starch, 1 Fruit, 2 Meat, 1 Milk, 1 Fat
LUNCH	**Hickory Grilled Chicken Sandwiches,** *page 198,* 1 serving Carrot sticks, ½ c Fresh fruit salad, ½ c	**Hickory Grilled Chicken Sandwiches,** *page 198,* 1 serving Low-fat potato chips, 1½ oz Carrot sticks, ½ c Fresh fruit salad, ½ c	**Hickory Grilled Chicken Sandwiches,** *page 198,* 1 serving Low-fat potato chips, 1½ oz Carrot sticks, ½ c Fresh fruit salad, ½ c
	1½ Starch, 1 Veg, 1½ Fruit, 3 Meat	3 Starch, 1 Veg, 1½ Fruit, 3 Meat, 1 Fat	3 Starch, 1 Veg, 1½ Fruit, 3 Meat, 1 Fat
DINNER	**Tomato-Basil Pizza,** *page 83,* 1 slice **Italian-Style Salad,** *page 145,* 1 serving Pear, 1	**Tomato-Basil Pizza,** *page 83,* 2 slices **Italian-Style Salad,** *page 145,* 1 serving	**Tomato-Basil Pizza,** *page 83,* 2 slices **Italian-Style Salad,** *page 145,* 1 serving
	2 Starch, 2 Veg, 1 Fruit, 2 Meat, 1 Fat	4 Starch, 3 Veg, 4 Meat, 2 Fat	4 Starch, 3 Veg, 4 Meat, 2 Fat
SNACK	Whole wheat bread, 1 slice Roast beef, 1 oz Mayonnaise, 1 tbls Mustard	Whole wheat bread, 2 slices Roast beef, 1 oz Mayonnaise, 1 tbls Mustard	Whole wheat bread, 2 slices Roast beef, 2 oz Mayonnaise, 1 tbls Mustard
	1 Starch, 1 Meat, 1 Fat	2 Starch, 1 Meat, 1 Fat	2 Starch, 2 Meat, 1 Fat

FRIDAY

	1500 calories	1800 calories	2000 calories
BREAKFAST	Bagel, 1 small Light cream cheese, 2 tbls Sliced strawberries, 1 c Fat-free yogurt, 8 oz	Bagel, 1 small Light cream cheese, 2 tbls Sliced strawberries, 1 c Fat-free yogurt, 8 oz	Bagel, 1½ small Light cream cheese, 2 tbls Sliced strawberries, 1 c Fat-free yogurt, 8 oz
	2 Starch, 1 Fruit, 1 Milk, 2 Fat	2 Starch, 1 Fruit, 1 Milk, 2 Fat	3 Starch, 1 Fruit, 1 Milk, 2 Fat
LUNCH	**Turkey Muffuletta Pitas,** *page 201,* 1 serving **Raspberry Smoothies,** *page 46,* 1 serving	**Turkey Muffuletta Pitas,** *page 201,* 2 serving **Raspberry Smoothies,** *page 46,* 1 serving	**Turkey Muffuletta Pitas,** *page 201,* 2 serving **Raspberry Smoothies,** *page 46,* 1 serving
	2 Starch, 1 Veg, 1 Fruit, 1 Meat	3 Starch, 2 Veg, 1 Fruit, 2 Meat	3 Starch, 2 Veg, 1 Fruit, 2 Meat
DINNER	**Cajun Catfish,** *page 62,* 1 serving Steamed rice, ½ c Steamed zucchini, ½ c French bread, 1 slice Light butter, 2 tbls Sliced peaches, ½ c	**Cajun Catfish,** *page 62,* 1 serving Steamed rice, 1 c Steamed zucchini, ½ c French bread, 1 slice Light butter, 2 tbls Sliced peaches, ½ c	**Cajun Catfish,** *page 62,* 1 serving Steamed rice, 1 c Steamed zucchini, 1 c French bread, 1 slice Light butter, 2 tbls Sliced peaches, ½ c
	2 Starch, 1 Veg, 1 Fruit, 4 Meat, 2 Fat	3 Starch, 1 Veg, 1 Fruit, 4 Meat, 2 Fat	3 Starch, 2 Veg, 1 Fruit, 4 Meat, 2 Fat
SNACK	Vanilla wafers, 5 Peanut butter, 1 tbls	Vanilla wafers, 10 Peanut butter, 1 tbls	Vanilla wafers, 10 Peanut butter, 2 tbls
	1 Starch, 1 Meat, 1 Fat	2 Starch, 1 Meat, 1 Fat	2 Starch, 2 Meat, 2 Fat

Abbreviations Key: **tbls** = tablespoon(s)   **tsp** = teaspoon(s)   **oz** = ounce(s)   **c** = cup(s)   **Veg** = Vegetable Exchange

SATURDAY

1500 calories	1800 calories	2000 calories
Cheese toast (2 slices whole wheat bread, 1 oz cheese) Sliced strawberries, 1 c Sugar-free cocoa, 1 c	Cheese toast (2 slices whole wheat bread, 1 oz cheese) Sliced strawberries, 1 c Sugar-free cocoa, 1 c	Cheese toast (2 slices whole wheat bread, 2 oz cheese) Instant grits, ½ c Sliced strawberries, 1 c Sugar-free cocoa, 1 c
2 Starch, 1 Fruit, 1 Meat, 1 Milk, 1 Fat	**2 Starch, 1 Fruit, 1 Meat, 1 Milk, 1 Fat**	**3 Starch, 1 Fruit, 2 Meat, 1 Milk, 2 Fat**
Salad Niçoise, *page 157,* 1 serving Crisp breadsticks, 4 Nectarine, 1	**Salad Niçoise,** *page 157,* 1 serving Crisp breadsticks, 4 Nectarine, 1 No added sugar ice cream, ½ c	**Salad Niçoise,** *page 157,* 1 serving Crisp breadsticks, 4 Nectarine, 1 No added sugar ice cream, ½ c
2 Starch, 1 Veg, 1 Fruit, 4 Meat	**3 Starch, 1 Veg, 1 Fruit, 4 Meat, 1 Fat**	**3 Starch, 1 Veg, 1 Fruit, 4 Meat, 1 Fat**
Szechuan Chicken and Vegetables, *page 120,* 1 serving Noodles, 1 c Peach, 1	**Szechuan Chicken and Vegetables,** *page 120,* 1 serving Noodles, 1 c **Easy Peach Ice Cream,** *page 49,* 1 serving	**Szechuan Chicken and Vegetables,** *page 120,* 1 serving Noodles, 1 c **Easy Peach Ice Cream,** *page 49,* 1 serving
2 Starch, 2 Veg, 1 Fruit, 3 Meat	**2½ Starch, 2 Veg, 1 Fruit, 3 Meat**	**2½ Starch, 2 Veg, 1 Fruit, 3 Meat**
Whole wheat bread, 1 slice Turkey, 1 oz Mayonnaise, 1 tbls Mustard	Whole wheat bread, 1 slice Turkey, 1 oz Mayonnaise, 1 tbls Mustard Fat-free milk, 1 c	Whole wheat bread, 2 slices Turkey, 2 oz Mayonnaise, 2 tbls Mustard
1 Starch, 1 Meat, 1 Fat	**1 Starch, 1 Meat, 1 Milk, 1 Fat**	**2 Starch, 2 Meat, 2 Fat**

SUNDAY

1500 calories	1800 calories	2000 calories
Egg Olé Burritos, *page 80,* 1 serving Grapefruit, 1 Fat free milk, 1 c	**Egg Olé Burritos,** *page 80,* 2 servings Grapefruit, ½ Fat free milk, 1 c	**Egg Olé Burritos,** *page 80,* 2 servings Grapefruit, ½ Fat free milk, 1 c
1½ Starch, 2 Fruit, 1 Meat, 1 Milk	**3 Starch, 1 Fruit, 2 Meat, 1 Milk**	**3 Starch, 1 Fruit, 2 Meat, 1 Milk**
Curry-Orange Chicken, *page 122,* 1 serving Steamed broccoli with cheese sauce, ½ c	**Curry-Orange Chicken,** *page 122,* 1 serving Steamed broccoli with cheese sauce, ½ c Canned crushed pineapple, ½ c	**Curry-Orange Chicken,** *page 122,* 1 serving Steamed broccoli with cheese sauce, 1 c Canned crushed pineapple, ½ c
3 Starch, 1 Veg, 2 Meat, 1 Fat	**3 Starch, 1 Veg, 1 Fruit, 2 Meat, 1 Fat**	**3 Starch, 2 Veg, 1 Fruit, 2 Meat, 2 Fat**
Meatless Chili, *page 89,* 1 serving Celery sticks with 2 tbls peanut butter Apple, 1	**Meatless Chili,** *page 89,* 1 serving Baked tortilla chips, 1 oz Celery sticks with 2 tbls peanut butter Apple, 1	**Meatless Chili,** *page 89,* 1 serving Baked tortilla chips, 1 oz Celery sticks with 2 tbls peanut butter Apple, 1
2 Starch, 1 Veg, 1 Fruit, 3 Meat, 2 Fat	**3 Starch, 1 Veg, 1 Fruit, 3 Meat, 2 Fat**	**3 Starch, 1 Veg, 1 Fruit, 3 Meat, 2 Fat**
Popped popcorn, 3 c Cheddar cheese, 1 oz	Popped popcorn, 6 c Cheddar cheese, 1 oz	Popped popcorn, 6 c Cheddar cheese, 2 oz
1 Starch, 1 Meat	**2 Starch, 1 Meat**	**2 Starch, 2 Meat**

sugar substitute guide

Sugar Substitute*	Description	Amount to equal ½ cup sugar
The following sugar substitutes are measured like sugar, so when you use them in recipes to replace sugar, use the same amount of substitute as you would use of sugar.		
DiabetiSweet	Contains a combination of acesulfame-K and isomalt; no aftertaste; looks like sugar; heat stable	½ cup
Equal Spoonful	Contains aspartame; no aftertaste; loses some sweetness in high heat	½ cup
Splenda	Contains sucralose, a modified sugar molecule that is not absorbed by the body; no aftertaste; extremely heat stable; also available in packets	½ cup
Sugar Twin	Contains saccharin; some aftertaste; heat stable	½ cup
These sugar substitutes are in more concentrated form, so you do not use as much of these as you would use of sugar in order to get the same sweetness.		
Equal for Recipes	Contains aspartame; no aftertaste; the bulk form of Equal packets; loses some sweetness in high heat	3½ teaspoons
Equal Packets	Contains aspartame; no aftertaste; same as Equal for Recipes (above), but in packets; loses some sweetness in high heat	12 packets
Sweet 'N Low	Contains saccharin; some aftertaste; available in bulk form or in packets; heat stable	1 tablespoon or 12 packets
Sweet One	Contains acesulfame-K; no aftertaste; heat stable	12 packets
Liquid sugar substitutes blend easily with other ingredients and work well in sauces and marinades.		
Sweet 'N Low	Contains saccharin; some aftertaste; heat stable	1 tablespoon
Sweet-10	Contains saccharin; some aftertaste; heat stable	1 tablespoon

*This list includes the sugar substitutes that we use most often in our Test Kitchens. It is not an inclusive list and is not meant as an endorsement of any particular product.

Appetizers & Beverages

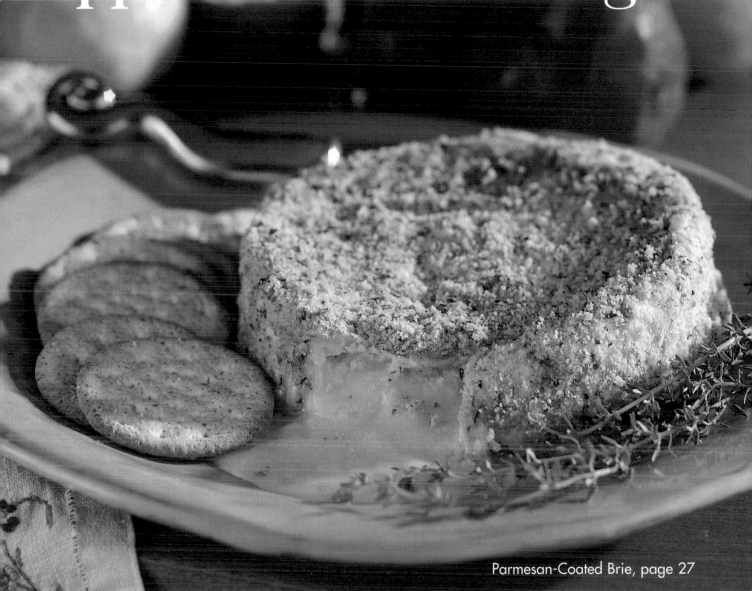

Parmesan-Coated Brie, page 27

Light Guacamole · Classic Onion Dip · Red Pepper Pesto Crostini

Garlic-Herb Cheese Spread · Parmesan-Coated Brie · Chicken Nacho Wedges

Hot Spiced Cheer · Black Currant-and-Raspberry Cooler · Mocha Smoothies

Prep: 10 minutes

Light Guacamole

1	large Anaheim chile (about 3 ounces)
2	green onions, cut into 2-inch pieces
2	garlic cloves, peeled and halved
2	large plum tomatoes, quartered
¾	cup peeled diced avocado (about 1 small)
½	cup tomatillo salsa
¼	cup cilantro sprigs
2	tablespoons fresh lemon or lime juice
½	teaspoon ground cumin
¼	teaspoon salt

Lime slices (optional)

Cut chile in half lengthwise; discard stem, seeds, and membranes.

Place chile, green onions, and garlic in a food processor; pulse 5 times or until coarsely chopped. Add tomato and next 6 ingredients; pulse 10 times until blended (mixture should be chunky). Spoon into a bowl; garnish with lime slices, if desired. Serve with low-fat tortilla chips (chips not included in analysis). **Yield:** 2 cups (serving size: ¼ cup).

Per Serving:

Calories 40	**Fiber** 1.3g
Fat 2.3g (sat 0.4g)	**Cholesterol** 0mg
Protein 0.8g	**Sodium** 79mg
Carbohydrate 4.3g	**Exchanges:** 1 Vegetable, ½ Fat

Here's a great dip to take to a Cinco de Mayo party. Don't forget the low-fat chips!

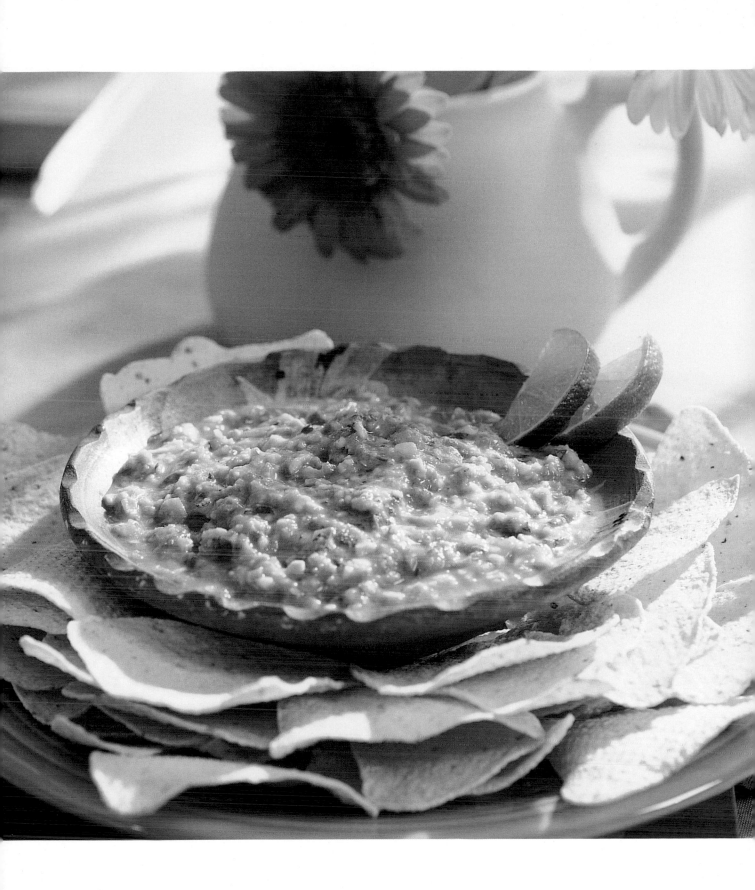

make *Ahead*

Prep: 10 minutes   Chill: 1 hour

Classic Onion Dip

1   (8-ounce) carton fat-free sour cream
½   cup finely chopped onion
2   teaspoons low-sodium soy sauce
¼   teaspoon garlic pepper

Combine all ingredients in a medium bowl; stir well. Cover and chill 1 hour. Serve with low-fat potato chips, crackers, or raw vegetables (chips, crackers, and vegetables not included in analysis). **Yield:** 1 cup (serving size: 1 tablespoon).

Per Serving:

Calories 12	**Fiber** 0.1g
Fat 0.0g (sat 0.0g)	**Cholesterol** 0mg
Protein 1.1g	**Sodium** 40mg
Carbohydrate 1.4g	**Exchange:** Free (up to 3 tablespoons)

Everybody enjoys good ol' onion dip! This one is made with fat-free sour cream and a splash of soy sauce. When you serve it with low-fat potato chips, no one will be able to resist!

Party On!

Don't let the temptation of party goodies wreck your diabetes control. Here's how to steer smoothly through any gathering.

Treats offered at holiday parties and special family celebrations may be tempting, but they can wreak havoc with blood sugars. Here are some tricks for sticking to diet plans during social occasions.

• Eat a regular meal before you go to a party. Then you won't be hungry and tempted to overindulge in snacks and sweets.

• Don't skip meals during the day to "save up" for over-eating at the party.

• Keep a glass of water or sugar-free soft drink in your hand at all times. It's harder to eat when one hand is busy.

• Don't stand next to the serving table all night. Move to another place in the room.

• Enjoy conversation. When your mouth is busy talking, it's not busy eating.

• Drink lots of water before a party. You'll feel full and be less tempted to snack.

• Offer to bring a low-fat, low-sugar dish to the party.

• Fill up on low-calorie, high-fiber foods, such as fresh vegetables and fruits. But go easy on the vegetable dip and cheese.

• If you must have something sweet, go ahead and have a little taste. Just allow for the extra carbohydrate in your meal plan.

• Keep the fat content of your regular meals especially low during the holidays to balance the extra fat from party foods.

• Share ideas for healthful treats as a holiday gift to your friends. Furnish them with healthy recipes as they plan holiday parties. Or go a step further and put together a booklet of healthy (and diabetes-friendly) recipes.

Party Picks:

Choose these low-fat, low-sugar party foods.

Fruits
Apple wedges
Grapes
Pear slices
Pineapple
Strawberries

Vegetables
Broccoli florets
Carrot sticks
Cauliflower
Celery sticks
Cherry tomatoes
Squash slices

Breads & Starches
Breadsticks
French bread
Low-fat potato chips
Low-fat tortilla chips
Melba rounds
Pita bread wedges
Plain crackers
Plain rolls
Pretzels

Meats, Poultry & Seafood
Lean roast beef
Pork tenderloin
Turkey
Boiled shrimp

Dips
Black bean dip
Salsa

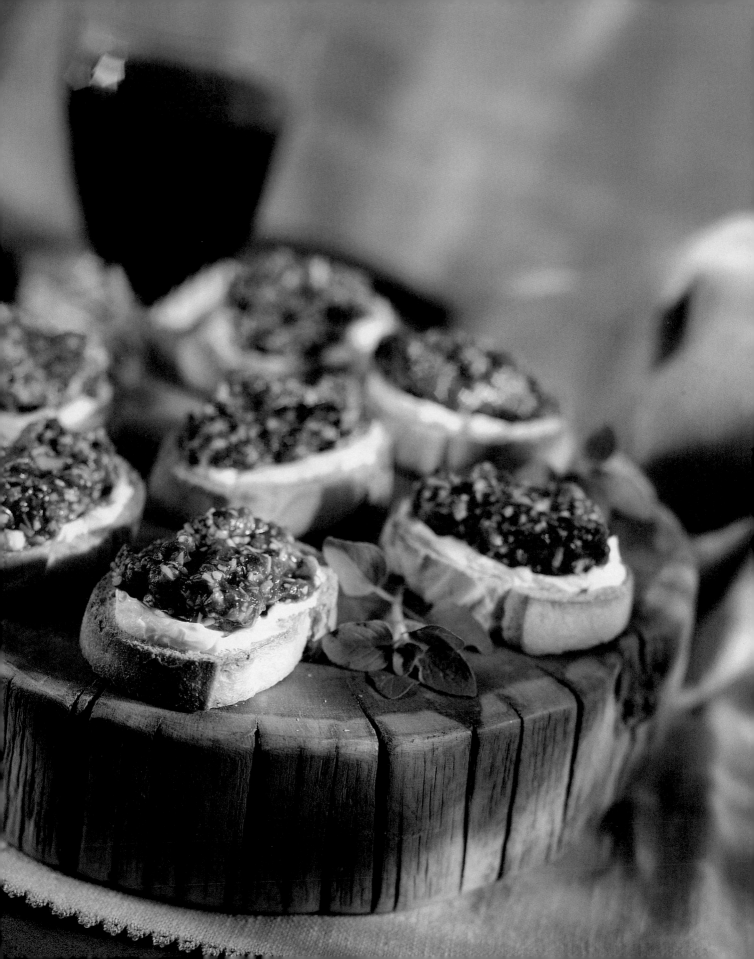

make *Ahead*

Prep: 5 minutes   Chill: 1 hour

Red Pepper Pesto Crostini

1   (7-ounce) jar roasted red pepper, drained and coarsely chopped
3   tablespoons freshly grated Parmesan cheese
1   tablespoon sliced almonds, toasted
2   teaspoons no-salt-added tomato paste
1   garlic clove, chopped
3   ounces fat-free cream cheese
16 (½-inch-thick) slices French bread baguette, toasted

Combine first 5 ingredients in a blender; process until smooth, stopping once to scrape down sides. Cover and chill at least 1 hour.

Spread cream cheese evenly on toast slices; top each with 1 tablespoon pepper mixture. **Yield:** 16 appetizers.

Per Appetizer:

Calories 86   Fiber 0.6g
Fat 1.2g (sat 0.3g)   Cholesterol 2mg
Protein 3.4g   Sodium 207mg
Carbohydrate 14.7g   Exchange: 1 Starch

This red pepper pesto adds zest to grilled fish, pasta, or a sandwich.

Prep: 12 minutes   Chill: 1 hour

Garlic-Herb Cheese Spread

1½   cups fat-free sour cream
½   cup light cream cheese
1   tablespoon minced fresh chives
2   teaspoons minced fresh parsley
½   teaspoon salt
½   teaspoon pepper
½   teaspoon minced bottled garlic

Combine sour cream and cream cheese in a bowl. Stir in chives and remaining ingredients; cover and chill at least 1 hour. Serve on bagel chips or toasted French bread (chips and bread not included in analysis). **Yield:** *2 cups (serving size: 1 tablespoon).*

Per Serving:

Calories 16

Fat 0.6g (sat 0.4g)

Protein 1.2g

Carbohydrate 1.1g

Fiber 0.0g

Cholesterol 2mg

Sodium 65mg

Exchange: Free (up to ¼ cup)

Here's a cheese spread that you can whip up and keep on hand for unexpected guests.

Prep: 10 minutes   Chill: 1 hour   Cook: 10 minutes

Parmesan-Coated Brie

1   large egg, lightly beaten
1   tablespoon water
¼   cup dry breadcrumbs
¼   cup grated fat-free Parmesan cheese
1½   teaspoons dried Italian seasoning
1   (15-ounce) round Brie cheese with herbs
Cooking spray
Fresh rosemary sprigs (optional)

Combine egg and water in a shallow dish. Combine breadcrumbs, Parmesan cheese, and seasoning in another shallow dish.

Dip Brie into egg mixture, turning to coat top and sides (do not coat bottom). Place Brie in breadcrumb mixture, turning to coat top and sides. Repeat procedure. Place on a baking sheet coated with cooking spray. Chill at least 1 hour.

Preheat oven to 375°.

Bake at 375° for 10 minutes. Garnish with rosemary, if desired. Serve with low-fat crackers or French baguette slices (crackers and bread not included in analysis). **Yield:** 15 appetizer servings.

Per Serving:

Calories 110	**Fiber** 0.1g
Fat 8.0g (sat 5.0g)	**Cholesterol** 28mg
Protein 6.4g	**Sodium** 228mg
Carbohydrate 2.9g	**Exchange:** 1 High-Fat Meat

(Photograph on page 19)

Prep: 17 minutes   Cook: 8 minutes

Chicken Nacho Wedges

Cooking spray
4   (8-inch) fat-free flour tortillas
1   cup finely chopped green bell pepper
¾   cup finely chopped red onion
1½   teaspoons ground cumin
1   (14½-ounce) can Mexican-style stewed tomatoes,
          undrained and chopped
1½   cups chopped cooked chicken breast
¼   cup minced fresh cilantro
1   cup (4 ounces) shredded reduced-fat Monterey Jack cheese

Preheat oven to 375°.

Arrange tortillas on a large baking sheet coated with cooking spray; set aside.

Coat a large nonstick skillet with cooking spray; place over medium heat until hot. Add green pepper and onion; sauté 5 minutes or until tender. Add cumin, and cook 1 minute. Add tomato; cook 3 minutes, stirring occasionally.

Spoon tomato mixture evenly over tortillas; top with chicken and cilantro. Sprinkle cheese evenly over chicken. Bake at 375° for 8 minutes or until tortillas are crisp. Cut each tortilla into 6 wedges. Serve immediately. **Yield:** 24 wedges.

Per Wedge:

Calories 57	**Fiber** 0.4g
Fat 1.4g (sat 0.6g)	**Cholesterol** 11mg
Protein 5.2g	**Sodium** 138mg
Carbohydrate 5.9g	**Exchanges:** ½ Starch, ½ Lean Meat

Prep: 5 minutes   Cook: 25 minutes

Hot Spiced Cheer

10 whole cloves
4   (3-inch) cinnamon sticks
4   pieces crystallized ginger, chopped
1   gallon apple juice
4   cups pineapple juice
2   cups orange juice
¼   cup fresh lemon juice
⅓   cup "measures-like-sugar" calorie-free sweetener
¼   teaspoon salt

Place first 3 ingredients on a double layer of cheesecloth. Gather edges of cheesecloth together; tie securely.

Combine cheesecloth bag, apple juice, and remaining ingredients in a large stockpot; bring to a boil. Reduce heat, and simmer 20 minutes. Discard cheesecloth bag. Serve warm. **Yield:** 22 (1-cup) servings.

Per Serving:

Calories 133	**Fiber** 0.3g
Fat 0.3g (sat 0.0g)	**Cholesterol** 0mg
Protein 0.4g	**Sodium** 33mg
Carbohydrate 33.0g	**Exchanges:** 2 Fruit

You'll be a popular host when you serve this hot fruity punch at holiday parties. Your friends with diabetes—and those who are trying to lose weight—can relax and enjoy, knowing it's not loaded with sugar.

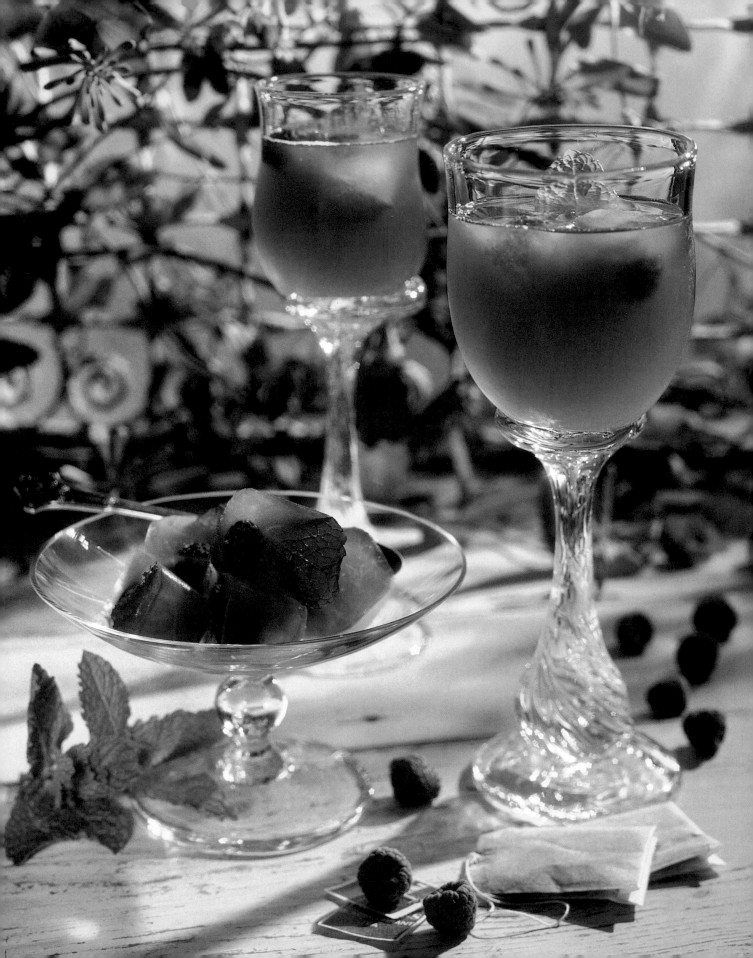

Prep: 15 minutes   Freeze: 1 hour

Black Currant-and-Raspberry Cooler

4½   cups apple-raspberry fruit juice blend, divided
14   raspberries
14   mint leaves
2½   cups water
4   black currant-flavored tea bags

Pour 1 cup fruit juice into an ice cube tray; place 1 raspberry and 1 mint leaf in each section of ice cube tray. Freeze until firm.

Bring water to a boil in a medium saucepan. Add tea bags; remove from heat. Cover and steep 10 minutes. Remove and discard tea bags.

Combine tea and 3½ cups fruit juice in a large pitcher. Cover and chill. Place frozen juice cubes in glasses; pour tea mixture over cubes. **Yield:** 6 (1-cup) servings.

Per Serving:

Calories 72	Fiber 0.5g
Fat 0.0g (sat 0.0g)	Cholesterol 0mg
Protein 0.1g	Sodium 18mg
Carbohydrate 18.4g	Exchange: 1 Fruit

The fruited ice cubes add an elegant and tasty touch to this beverage. And they're so easy to make!

Prep: 10 minutes

Mocha Smoothies

3	cups fat-free milk
1	cup water
½	cup sugar-free chocolate-flavored syrup (such as Sweet 'N Low)
2	to 3 teaspoons instant coffee granules
1	teaspoon vanilla extract
1	quart vanilla no-sugar-added, fat-free ice cream

Combine first 5 ingredients in a blender; process until blended.

Pour half of chocolate mixture into a bowl. Add half of ice cream to chocolate mixture in blender; process until smooth. Pour ice cream mixture into a 2-quart pitcher.

Combine remaining chocolate mixture and remaining ice cream in blender; process until smooth. Add to ice cream mixture in pitcher, and stir. Serve immediately. **Yield:** 8 (1-cup) servings.

Per Serving:

Calories 124	**Fiber** 0.5g
Fat 0.2g (sat 0.1g)	**Cholesterol** 2mg
Protein 7.2g	**Sodium** 125mg
Carbohydrate 25.1g	**Exchanges:** 1 Starch, ½ Skim Milk

If you have coffee left over from breakfast, use 1 cup of cold, strong coffee instead of water and instant coffee granules.

Breads

Coconut Muffins, page 43

Prep: 7 minutes   Cook: 15 minutes

Tomato-Parmesan Flatbread

2   tablespoons dried tomato bits (packed without oil)
1½ tablespoons fat-free Caesar Italian dressing
1   (11.3-ounce) can refrigerated dinner rolls
2   tablespoons grated garlic-herb Parmesan cheese blend
Cooking spray

Preheat oven to 375°.

Combine tomato bits and dressing in a small bowl; let mixture stand 5 minutes.

Separate dough into rolls. Roll each piece into a 4-inch round. Place rounds on a baking sheet coated with cooking spray.

Brush rounds evenly with tomato mixture, and sprinkle evenly with Parmesan cheese blend. Bake at 375° for 15 minutes or until golden. **Yield:** 8 servings (serving size: 1 flatbread).

Per Serving:

Calories 129	**Fiber** 0.3g
Fat 2.1g (sat 0.0g)	**Cholesterol** 0mg
Protein 4.3g	**Sodium** 393mg
Carbohydrate 20.8g	**Exchanges:** 1½ Starch, ½ Fat

You can make your own garlic-herb Parmesan cheese by combining 2 tablespoons regular grated Parmesan cheese, ½ teaspoon dried Italian seasoning, and ⅛ teaspoon garlic powder.

Date Delights

1   (8-ounce) can refrigerated reduced-fat crescent roll dough
2   tablespoons light butter, melted and divided
8   packets calorie-free sweetener
1   tablespoon ground cinnamon
8   whole pitted dates
Cooking spray
Additional ground cinnamon (optional)

Preheat oven to 375°.

Separate rolls into 8 triangles; brush triangles evenly with 1 tablespoon melted butter. Sprinkle 1 packet sweetener on each triangle. Sprinkle triangles evenly with 1 tablespoon cinnamon.

Place 1 date on each triangle; pinch dough around date, sealing all edges. Place each in a muffin cup coated with cooking spray. Brush tops with 1 tablespoon butter; sprinkle lightly with additional cinnamon, if desired.

Bake at 375° for 13 to 15 minutes or until golden. Remove from muffin cups, and serve immediately. **Yield:** 8 muffins.

Per Muffin:

Calories 137	Fiber 0.9g
Fat 6.1g (sat 2.0g)	Cholesterol 5mg
Protein 2.5g	Sodium 251mg
Carbohydrate 18.3g	Exchanges: 1 Starch, 1 Fat

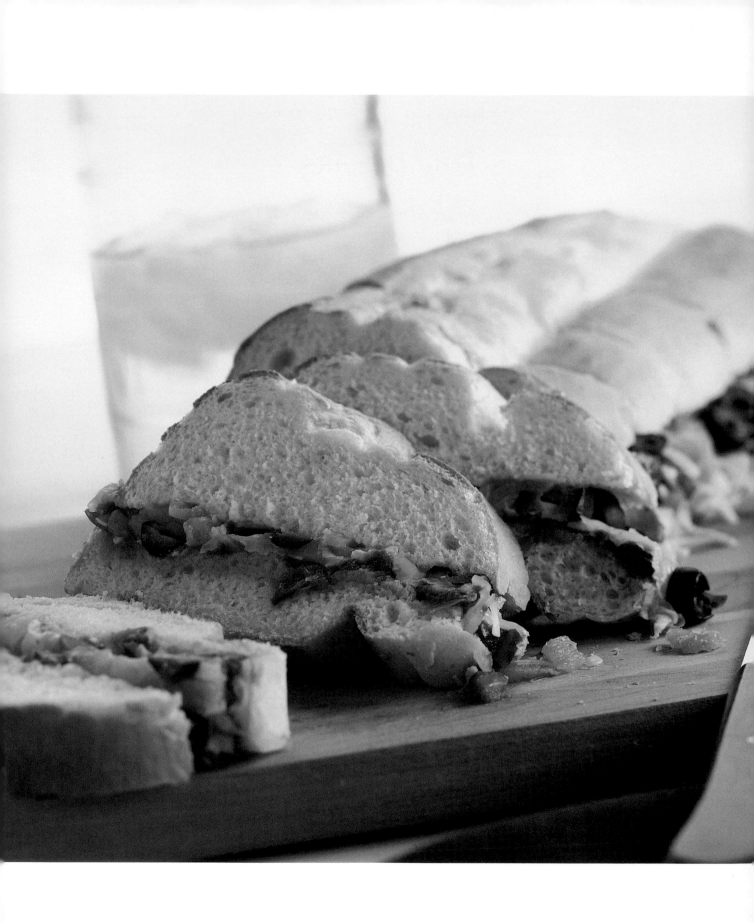

Prep: 5 minutes   Cook: 20 minutes

Stuffed Tex-Mex Loaf

1   cup bottled salsa
1   (16-ounce) loaf French bread, cut in half lengthwise
1   cup (4 ounces) preshredded reduced-fat Mexican cheese blend
        (such as Sargento Light)
1   (4.5-ounce) can chopped green chiles, drained
1   (2¼-ounce) can sliced ripe olives, drained

Preheat oven to 400°.

Spread salsa over bottom half of bread. Top with cheese, chiles, olives, and top half of bread.

Wrap in foil; bake at 400° for 20 minutes or until cheese melts and bread is toasted. Let stand 5 minutes. Cut into slices, using a serrated knife. **Yield:** 10 servings (serving size: 1 slice).

Per Serving:

Calories 168	Fiber 2.0g
Fat 4.0g (sat 1.6g)	Cholesterol 4mg
Protein 7.6g	Sodium 526mg
Carbohydrate 26.0g	Exchanges: 1½ Starch, 1 Fat

Blueberry Pancakes

1	cup all-purpose flour
2	teaspoons baking powder
¼	teaspoon baking soda
¼	teaspoon salt
1	tablespoon sugar
1⅓	cups low-fat buttermilk
¼	cup egg substitute
1	tablespoon vegetable oil
½	cup fresh or frozen blueberries

Cooking spray

Combine first 5 ingredients in a large bowl. Combine buttermilk, egg substitute, and oil; add to dry ingredients, stirring just until moist. Stir in blueberries.

Pour ¼ cup batter per pancake onto a hot griddle or large skillet coated with cooking spray. Cook until tops are bubbly and edges look cooked; turn and cook other sides. Repeat with remaining batter. **Yield:** 12 pancakes (serving size: 2 pancakes).

Per Serving:

Calories 143	**Fiber** 0.9g
Fat 2.9g (sat 0.6g)	**Cholesterol** 2mg
Protein 5.8g	**Sodium** 402mg
Carbohydrate 23.6g	**Exchanges:** 1½ Starch, ½ Fat

Prep: 5 minutes   Cook: 30 minutes

Skillet Bread

Cooking spray
¾ cup uncooked instant farina (such as Instant Cream of Wheat)
¾ cup self-rising flour
2 teaspoons baking powder
1 cup low-fat buttermilk
2 tablespoons vegetable oil
1 large egg

Preheat oven to 450°.

Coat an 8-inch cast iron skillet with cooking spray.

Combine farina, flour, and baking powder in a bowl; make a well in center of mixture. Combine buttermilk, oil, and egg; add to dry ingredients, stirring just until moist. Spoon batter into skillet. Bake at 450° for 30 minutes or until golden. Cut into 8 wedges. **Yield:** 8 servings.

Per Serving:

Calories 156	Fiber 0.9g
Fat 4.7g (sat 0.7g)	Cholesterol 28mg
Protein 4.8g	Sodium 321mg
Carbohydrate 23.4g	Exchanges: 1½ Starch, 1 Fat

Prep: 12 minutes   Cook: 15 minutes

Pecan Cornbread

⅓   cup finely chopped lean country ham (about 2 ounces)
1   (6.5-ounce) package golden corn muffin and bread mix (such as
        Betty Crocker)
½   cup fat-free milk
¼   cup coarsely chopped pecans, toasted
¼   cup egg substitute

Preheat oven to 425°.

Place an 8-inch cast iron skillet over medium-high heat until hot.
Add ham, and sauté 2 minutes or until lightly browned. Place ham
in a large bowl. Keep skillet hot.

Add muffin mix and remaining 3 ingredients to ham, stirring
just until moist. Pour batter into preheated skillet. Bake at 425°
for 15 minutes or until lightly browned. Cut into 8 wedges.
Yield: 8 servings.

Per Serving:

Calories 139	**Fiber** 0.3g
Fat 5.0g (sat 0.6g)	**Cholesterol** 6mg
Protein 5.0g	**Sodium** 358mg
Carbohydrate 20.0g	**Exchanges:** 1½ Starch, 1 Fat

If you don't have an iron skillet, use an 8-inch
round cake pan or an 8-inch square baking
pan, and don't preheat the pan.

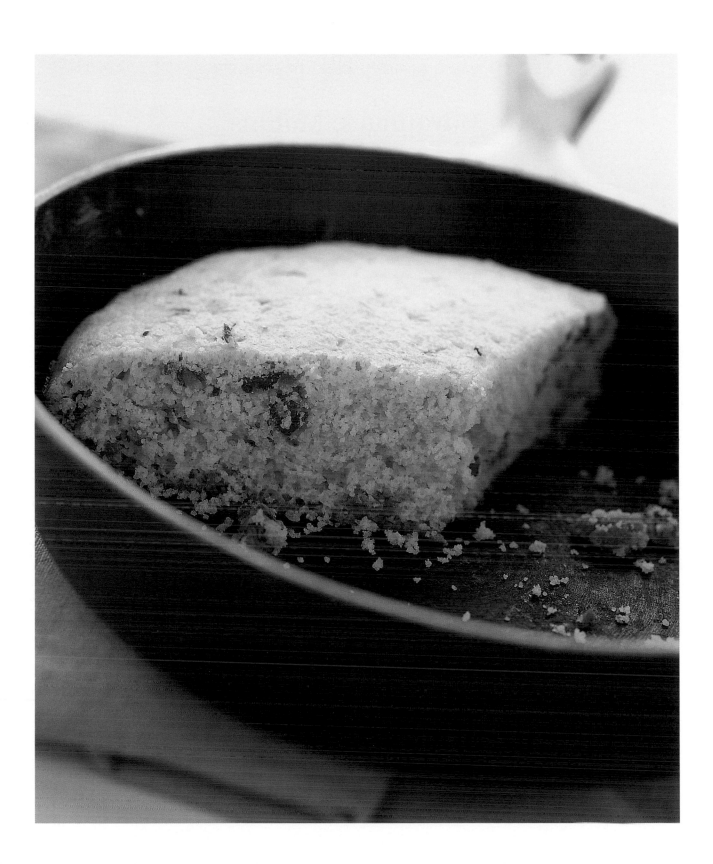

Prep: 5 minutes   Cook: 15 minutes

Mayonnaise Muffins

1   cup self-rising flour
½   cup 2% low-fat milk
¼   cup low-fat mayonnaise
Cooking spray

Preheat oven to 400°.

Combine all ingredients except cooking spray, stirring just until flour is moist. Spoon into muffin cups coated with cooking spray, filling two-thirds full.

Bake at 400° for 15 minutes or until lightly browned. Remove muffins from pan immediately. **Yield:** 6 muffins.

Per Muffin:

Calories 103	**Fiber** 0.6g
Fat 1.3g (sat 0.3g)	**Cholesterol** 2mg
Protein 3.0g	**Sodium** 385mg
Carbohydrate 19.6g	**Exchange:** 1 Starch

Only 4 ingredients and 5 minutes of work, and you've got tasty, tender low-fat muffins. And for smaller households, a half-dozen muffins is just the right amount!

Prep: 10 minutes   Cook: 19 minutes

Coconut Muffins

2   cups all-purpose flour
⅓   cup sugar
2   teaspoons baking powder
¼   teaspoon salt
¼   cup flaked sweetened coconut
1   (8-ounce) carton vanilla low-fat yogurt
¼   cup vegetable oil
¼   teaspoon coconut extract
1   large egg, lightly beaten
1   large egg white, lightly beaten
Cooking spray

Preheat oven to 400°.

Combine first 5 ingredients in a large bowl; make a well in center of mixture. Combine yogurt and next 4 ingredients; add to dry ingredients, stirring just until moist. Spoon into muffin cups coated with cooking spray, filling three-fourths full.

Bake at 400° for 19 to 20 minutes or until lightly browned. Remove muffins from pan immediately. **Yield:** 12 muffins.

Per Muffin:

Calories 169	**Fiber** 0.6g
Fat 5.9g (sat 1.1g)	**Cholesterol** 19mg
Protein 4.0g	**Sodium** 157mg
Carbohydrate 25.1g	**Exchanges:** 1½ Starch, 1 Fat

(Photograph on page 33)

PB&J Muffins

1½ cups all-purpose flour
2   teaspoons baking powder
½   teaspoon salt
¼   cup packed light brown sugar
⅔   cup fat-free milk
½   cup chunky reduced-fat peanut butter
½   cup egg substitute
Cooking spray
¼   cup plus 2 tablespoons fruit spread (such as Polaner All Fruit)

Preheat oven to 375°.

Combine first 4 ingredients in a large bowl; make a well in center of mixture. Combine milk, peanut butter, and egg substitute in a blender; process until blended. Add to dry ingredients, stirring just until moist.

Spoon batter into paper-lined muffin cups coated with cooking spray, filling about one-half full. Spread batter up sides of each muffin cup. Place 1½ teaspoons fruit spread in center of batter in each muffin cup; cover fruit spread completely with enough batter to fill each muffin cup three-fourths full. Bake at 375° for 18 to 20 minutes or until golden. Remove muffins from pan immediately, and serve warm. **Yield:** 12 muffins.

Per Muffin:

Calories 161	**Fiber** 0.4g
Fat 4.2g (sat 0.9g)	**Cholesterol** 0mg
Protein 5.6g	**Sodium** 195mg
Carbohydrate 25.8g	**Exchanges:** 1½ Starch, 1 Fat

Desserts

Crispy Peanut Butterscotch Pie, page 60

Prep: 5 minutes

Raspberry Smoothies

1½ cups fresh or frozen raspberries
1½ cups frozen reduced-calorie whipped topping, thawed
1   (8-ounce) carton lemon low-fat yogurt

Combine all ingredients in a blender. Add ice cubes to reach 4-cup level. Process until smooth. Serve immediately. **Yield:** 4 (1-cup) servings.

Per Serving:

Calories 144	**Fiber** 3.1g
Fat 0.7g (sat 0.0g)	**Cholesterol** 0mg
Protein 2.5g	**Sodium** 52mg
Carbohydrate 30.8g	**Exchanges:** 1 Starch, 1 Fruit

Strawberry Smoothies: Use 1½ cups sliced strawberries instead of raspberries, and proceed with recipe as directed.

Blueberry Smoothies: Use 1½ cups blueberries instead of raspberries, and proceed with recipe as directed.

Peach Smoothies: Use 1½ cups fresh or frozen sliced peaches instead of raspberries, use vanilla low-fat yogurt instead of lemon, and proceed with recipe as directed.

Prep: 15 minutes

Blueberry Sauce

2   tablespoons cornstarch
1¼   cups water, divided
2   cups blueberries
4   teaspoons "measures-like-sugar" calorie-free sweetener
1   teaspoon lemon juice

Combine cornstarch and ¼ cup water.

Combine blueberries and 1 cup water in a saucepan. Cook over medium-high heat 7 minutes or until blueberries are soft. Reduce heat to low, and add cornstarch mixture. Cook 1 minute or until thick.

Remove from heat, and cool slightly. Add sweetener and lemon juice; stir well. **Yield:** 2½ cups (serving size: ¼ cup).

Per Serving:

Calories 29
Fat 0.1g (sat 0.0g)
Protein 0.2g
Carbohydrate 7.2g

Fiber 0.8g
Cholesterol 0mg
Sodium 2mg
Exchange: ½ Fruit

For a summery treat, spoon this fruity sauce over no sugar added ice cream, angel food cake, or low-fat pound cake.

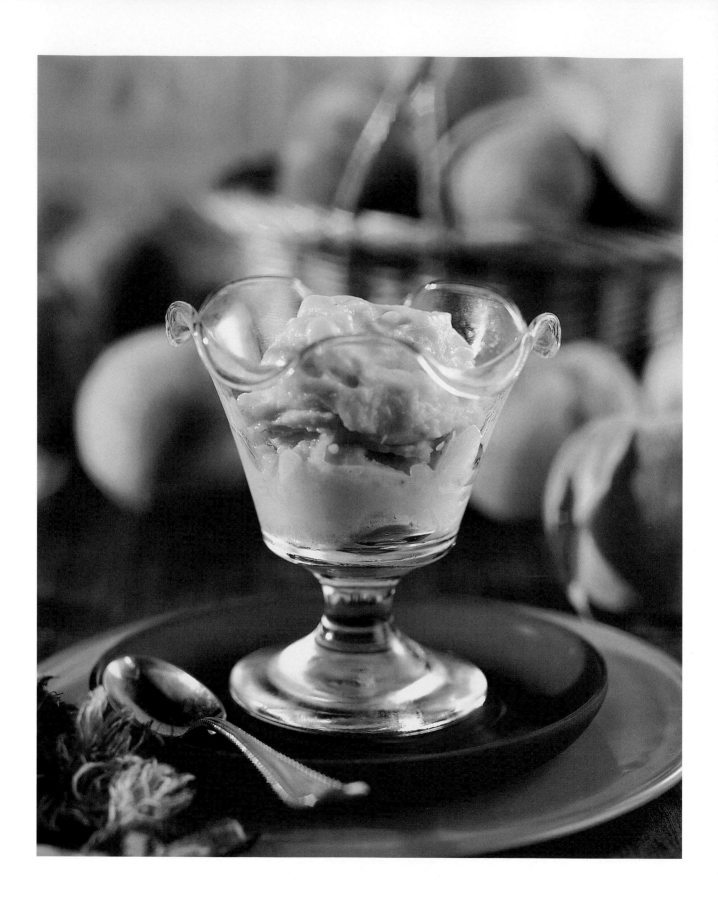

Prep: 12 minutes

Easy Peach Ice Cream

1   (1-pound) package frozen peaches
1½ cups sliced ripe banana (about 2)
1   cup vanilla low-fat, no sugar added ice cream
½   cup thawed orange juice concentrate
¼   cup "measures-like-sugar" calorie-free sweetener
¾   teaspoon coconut extract or ½ teaspoon almond extract

Combine all ingredients in a food processor; process until smooth. Serve immediately, or freeze, covered, in an airtight freezer-safe container until ready to serve. **Yield:** 9 (½-cup) servings.

Per Serving:

Calories 101	**Fiber** 1.7g
Fat 0.2g (sat 0.1g)	**Cholesterol** 0mg
Protein 1.3g	**Sodium** 6mg
Carbohydrate 25.0g	**Exchanges:** ½ Starch, 1 Fruit

Easy Strawberry Ice Cream: Use a 1-pound package frozen unsweetened strawberries instead of peaches and ¾ teaspoon vanilla extract instead of coconut extract.

superQuick

Nectarine Melba Sundaes

¼   cup raspberry spread (such as Polaner All Fruit)
2   tablespoons water
1   cup raspberries
2   cups thinly sliced unpeeled nectarines
2   cups vanilla fat-free, no sugar added ice cream

Combine raspberry spread and water in a small saucepan; bring to a boil over medium heat, stirring until smooth. Remove from heat; add raspberries, and stir gently.

Arrange nectarine slices evenly on 4 dessert plates; top each serving with ½ cup ice cream. Spoon raspberry mixture evenly over ice cream. **Yield:** 4 servings.

Per Serving:

Calories 135	**Fiber** 3.2g
Fat 0.5g (sat 0.0g)	**Cholesterol** 0mg
Protein 2.6g	**Sodium** 29mg
Carbohydrate 31.5g	**Exchanges:** 1 Starch, 1 Fruit

These sundaes are also delicious with sliced, peeled peaches instead of nectarines.

Blender Custard Cups

3   cups hot water
1   cup egg substitute
1   cup instant nonfat dry milk powder
¼   cup "measures-like-sugar" calorie-free sweetener
2   tablespoons sugar
1   tablespoon vanilla extract
¼   teaspoon salt
Ground nutmeg (optional)

Preheat oven to 325°.

Combine first 7 ingredients in a blender; process until smooth. Pour into 8 (6-ounce) custard cups. Sprinkle with nutmeg, if desired.

Set custard cups in a 13 x 9-inch baking pan; add hot water to pan to depth of 1 inch. Bake, uncovered, at 325° for 40 minutes. Serve custard warm or cold. **Yield:** 8 servings.

Per Serving:

Calories 82	**Fiber** 0.0g
Fat 0.1g (sat 0.0g)	**Cholesterol** 2mg
Protein 6.0g	**Sodium** 183mg
Carbohydrate 14.3g	**Exchange:** 1 Starch

Prep: 20 minutes

Tiramisu

½   cup strongly brewed chocolate-flavored coffee
3   tablespoons "measures-like-sugar" calorie-free sweetener, divided
3   tablespoons liquid fat-free hazelnut-flavored nondairy coffee
        creamer
½   cup tub-style light cream cheese, softened
¾   cup frozen fat-free whipped topping, thawed
½   (13.6-ounce) loaf fat-free pound cake, cut into 10 slices
Unsweetened cocoa (optional)

Combine coffee and 1 tablespoon sweetener. Spoon 2 tablespoons mixture into a medium bowl; set remaining mixture aside.

Add remaining sweetener and creamer to 2 tablespoons coffee mixture in bowl, stirring until sweetener dissolves. Add cream cheese; beat with a mixer at medium speed until smooth. Fold in whipped topping.

Place 1 cake slice in each of 5 wineglasses or custard cups. Brush cake generously with half of reserved coffee mixture. Spread cheese mixture evenly over cake. Top with remaining cake slices. Gently press slices into glasses. Brush cake with remaining coffee mixture. Sprinkle evenly with cocoa, if desired. **Yield:** 5 servings.

Per Serving:

Calories 229	**Fiber** 0.4g
Fat 4.5g (sat 2.9g)	**Cholesterol** 12mg
Protein 4.6g	**Sodium** 258mg
Carbohydrate 38.9g	**Exchanges:** 2½ Starch, 1 Fat

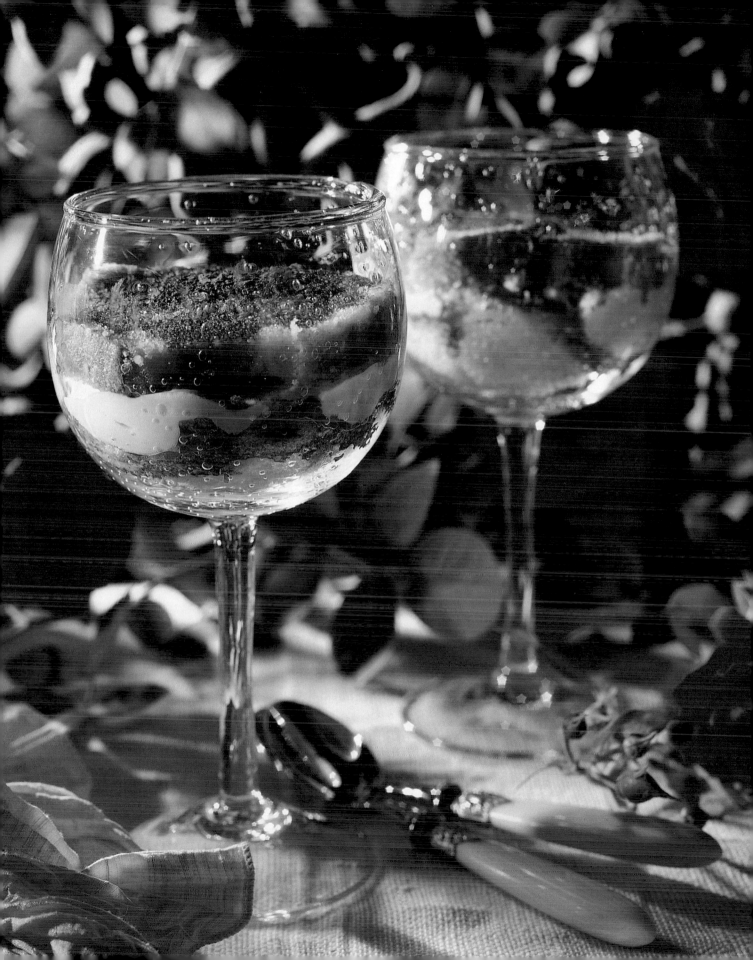

Prep: 15 minutes   Cook: 12 minutes

Banana Split Cake

1   (8-ounce) package white sugar-free, low-fat cake mix
Cooking spray
1   (1.5-ounce) package sugar-free vanilla instant pudding mix
3   cups fat-free milk
1   (20-ounce) can no sugar added cherry pie filling
1   (15-ounce) can pineapple tidbits in juice, drained
1   (16-ounce) package frozen unsweetened whole strawberries,
        thawed and sliced
3   large ripe bananas, sliced
1   (16-ounce) container frozen reduced-calorie whipped topping, thawed
¾   cup chopped walnuts
¼   cup sugar-free chocolate syrup (such as Sweet 'N Low)

Preheat oven to 350°.

Prepare cake mix according to package directions. Pour batter into
a 13 x 9-inch baking pan coated with cooking spray. Bake at 350°
for 12 minutes; cool slightly.

Prepare pudding according to package directions using 3 cups
fat-free milk. Spread pudding over cake. Top with pie filling,
pineapple, strawberries, and bananas. Top fruit with whipped
topping. Sprinkle with walnuts, and drizzle with chocolate syrup.
Yield: 18 servings (serving size: 2 x 3-inch piece).

Per Serving:

Calories 202	**Fiber** 1.8g
Fat 4.7g (sat 0.7g)	**Cholesterol** 1mg
Protein 3.4g	**Sodium** 96mg
Carbohydrate 39.7g	**Exchanges:** 1 Starch, 1½ Fruit, 1 Fat

(Photograph on cover)

Prep: 5 minutes   Cook: 9 minutes per batch

Angel Food Puffs

½   cup orange-flavored sugar-free carbonated beverage
¼   teaspoon almond extract
1   (16-ounce) package angel food cake mix
Cooking spray

Preheat oven to 350°.

Combine first 3 ingredients in a large bowl. Beat with a mixer at medium speed until smooth. Drop batter by heaping tablespoons onto baking sheets coated with cooking spray.

Bake at 350° for 9 minutes or until lightly browned. Remove from baking sheets immediately, and cool on wire racks.
Yield: 28 cookies.

Per Cookie:

Calories 61	Fiber 0.1g
Fat 0.1g (sat 0.0g)	Cholesterol 0mg
Protein 1.4g	Sodium 119mg
Carbohydrate 13.8g	Exchange: 1 Starch

(Photograph on page 1)

> You can change the flavor of these light, chewy cookies by using any other flavored sugar-free carbonated beverage. Try strawberry or lemon-lime for starters.

Orange Cookies

1½ cups all-purpose flour
1   teaspoon baking powder
¾   cup "measures-like-sugar" calorie-free sweetener
2   teaspoons grated orange peel
¼   teaspoon salt
⅛   teaspoon ground nutmeg
½   cup reduced-calorie margarine (with at least 70% oil)
⅓   cup chopped raisins
¼   cup egg substitute
1   tablespoon orange juice
Cooking spray

Preheat oven to 375°.

Combine first 6 ingredients in a large bowl. Cut in margarine with a pastry blender until mixture resembles coarse meal; stir in raisins. Stir in egg substitute and orange juice.

Drop dough by level teaspoons onto baking sheets coated with cooking spray. Bake at 375° for 13 minutes or until lightly browned. Remove from baking sheets immediately, and cool on wire racks. **Yield:** 29 cookies.

Per Cookie:

Calories 63	**Fiber** 0.3g
Fat 1.6g (sat 0.3g)	**Cholesterol** 0mg
Protein 0.9g	**Sodium** 80mg
Carbohydrate 11.4g	**Exchange:** 1 Starch

Ice Cream Torte

⅔   cup graham cracker crumbs (9 squares)
2   tablespoons reduced-calorie margarine, melted
Cooking spray
1   cup chocolate fat-free, no sugar added ice cream, softened
1   cup vanilla fat-free, no sugar added ice cream, softened
1   ounce sugar-free milk chocolate candy bar, melted

Combine graham cracker crumbs and margarine in a small bowl. Firmly press crumb mixture evenly into bottom of a 7-inch springform pan coated with cooking spray.

Spoon chocolate ice cream into crust; cover and freeze until set. Spoon vanilla ice cream over chocolate; cover and freeze until set.

Drizzle melted chocolate candy over ice cream, and cut into 6 wedges. **Yield:** 6 servings.

Per Serving:

Calories 151	**Fiber** 0.0g
Fat 5.1g (sat 1.2g)	**Cholesterol** 0.8mg
Protein 3.7g	**Sodium** 157mg
Carbohydrate 24.5g	**Exchanges:** 1½ Starch, 1 Fat

To melt the sugar-free chocolate candy, place candy in a small microwave-safe dish, and microwave at HIGH 1 minute and 30 seconds, stirring after 1 minute.

Turtle Pie

4   cups chocolate low-fat, no sugar added ice cream, softened
½   cup fat-free caramel topping, divided
1   (6-ounce) reduced-fat graham cracker crust
⅔   cup frozen fat-free whipped topping, thawed
2   tablespoons chopped pecans, toasted

Place an extra-large bowl in freezer for at least 5 minutes. Spoon ice cream into chilled bowl; stir in ¼ cup caramel topping. Spoon ice cream mixture into pie crust; cover and freeze 2½ hours or until firm.

Place pie in refrigerator to soften 10 to 15 minutes before serving.

Heat ¼ cup caramel topping according to label directions. Cut pie into 10 wedges, and top evenly with whipped topping. Drizzle evenly with warm caramel topping, and sprinkle with pecans.
Yield: 10 servings.

Per Serving:

Calories 178	**Fiber** 0.1g
Fat 3.9g (sat 0.5g)	**Cholesterol** 0mg
Protein 3.9g	**Sodium** 131mg
Carbohydrate 33.0g	**Exchanges:** 2 Starch

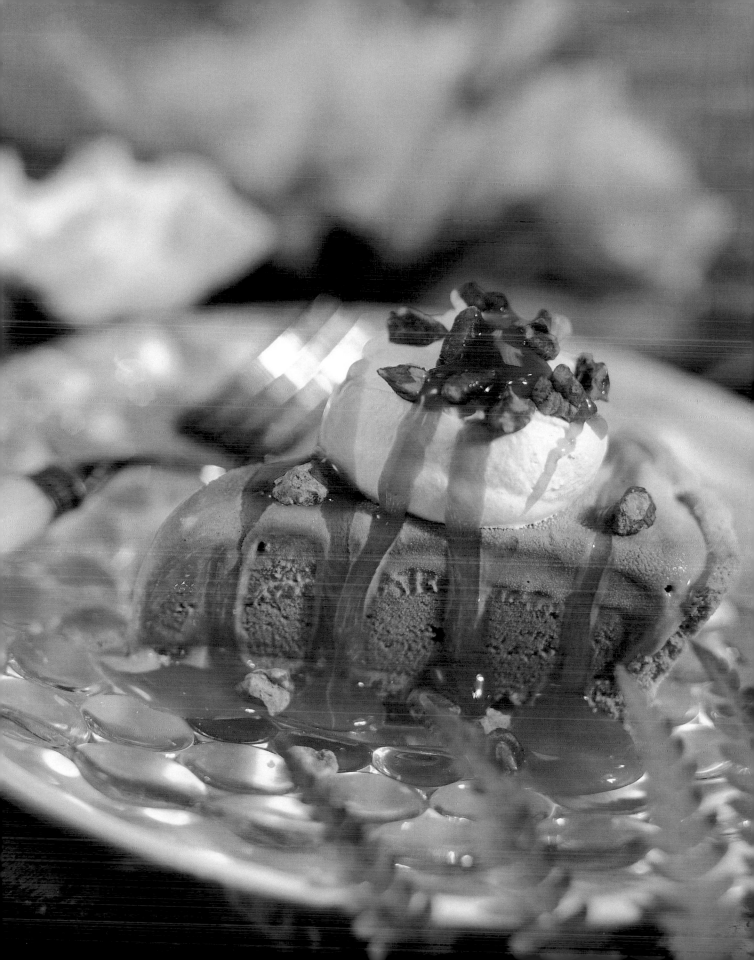

Crispy Peanut Butterscotch Pie

¼   cup creamy peanut butter
1   tablespoon honey
1½   cups oven-toasted rice cereal (such as Rice Krispies)
1   (1-ounce) package sugar-free butterscotch instant pudding mix
2   cups fat-free milk
1½   cups frozen fat-free whipped topping, thawed and divided
Ground cinnamon (optional)
Additional oven-toasted rice cereal (optional)

Combine peanut butter and honey in a medium microwave-safe bowl; microwave at HIGH 30 seconds, stirring until mixture melts. Stir in rice cereal. Using wax paper, press cereal mixture into bottom of an 8-inch round cake pan.

Prepare pudding mix according to package directions, using 2 cups fat-free milk; fold in 1 cup whipped topping. Spoon pudding mixture into prepared pan. Cover and freeze until firm. Let pie stand at room temperature 15 minutes before serving. Cut pie into 6 wedges, and top evenly with remaining whipped topping. If desired, sprinkle with ground cinnamon and additional cereal. **Yield:** 6 servings.

Per Serving:

Calories 149	**Fiber** 0.7g
Fat 5.0g (sat 0.9g)	**Cholesterol** 0mg
Protein 4.0g	**Sodium** 375mg
Carbohydrate 21.2g	**Exchanges:** 1½ Starch, 1 Fat

(Photograph on page 45)

Fish & Shellfish

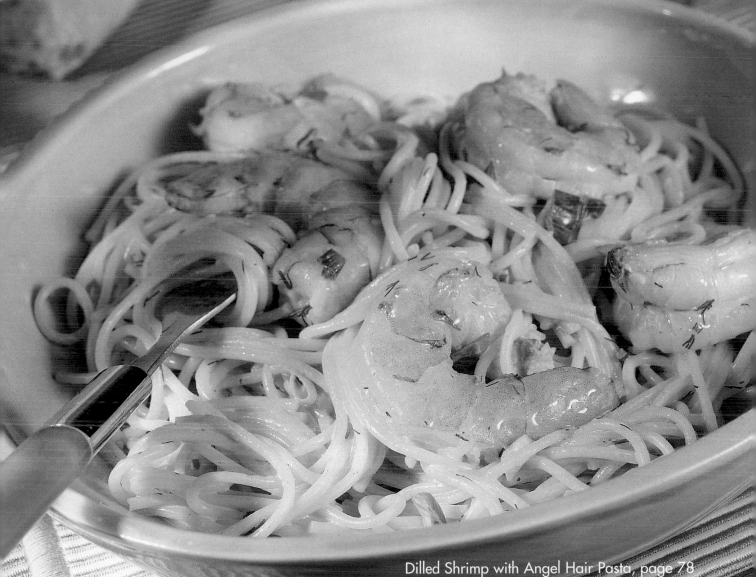

Dilled Shrimp with Angel Hair Pasta, page 78

Cajun Catfish • Grilled Halibut with Lemon Sauce • Greek-Style Orange Roughy
Lemon-Dill Fish Fillets • Spicy Lemon Red Snapper • Salmon with Pineapple Salsa
Grilled Salmon with Teriyaki Sauce • Grilled Tuna with Herbed Mayonnaise
Tuna with Tapenade • Tuna Casserole • Curried Sea Scallops
Shrimp with Feta • Dilled Shrimp with Angel Hair Pasta

Prep: 5 minutes   Cook: 10 minutes

Cajun Catfish

4   (6-ounce) farm-raised catfish fillets
1   tablespoon fresh lemon juice
4   teaspoons Cajun seasoning
Cooking spray
Lemon wedges (optional)

Preheat broiler.

Brush both sides of fillets with lemon juice, and sprinkle with seasoning. Place fish on a broiler pan coated with cooking spray. Broil 5 minutes on each side or until fish flakes easily when tested with a fork. Serve with lemon wedges, if desired. **Yield:** 4 servings.

Per Serving:

Calories 204	**Fiber** 0.4g
Fat 7.5g (sat 1.7g)	**Cholesterol** 99mg
Protein 31.2g	**Sodium** 249mg
Carbohydrate 1.5g	**Exchanges:** 4 Very Lean Meat

You can turn any kind of white fish into a Cajun treat. The only thing that might vary with a different kind of fish is the cooking time: allow about 7 to 9 minutes total cooking time per inch of thickness, measuring at the thickest part.

Prep: 8 minutes   Cook: 12 minutes

Grilled Halibut with Lemon Sauce

¾   cup fat-free, less-sodium chicken broth
¼   cup fresh lemon juice
1   tablespoon cornstarch
1   tablespoon minced fresh parsley
½   teaspoon salt
¼   teaspoon dried oregano
¼   teaspoon dried rosemary
Cooking spray
8   (6-ounce) halibut fillets

Combine first 3 ingredients in a small saucepan. Bring to a boil; cook 1 minute, stirring constantly. Remove from heat. Stir in parsley, salt, oregano, and rosemary; keep warm.

Prepare grill.

Place fish on grill rack coated with cooking spray; cover and grill 6 minutes on each side or until fish flakes easily when tested with a fork. Serve with warm sauce. **Yield:** 8 servings.

Per Serving:

Calories 197	Fiber 0.0g
Fat 4.2g (sat 0.6g)	Cholesterol 80mg
Protein 35.6g	Sodium 251mg
Carbohydrate 1.7g	Exchanges: 5 Very Lean Meat

Prep: 15 minutes   Cook: 20 minutes

Greek-Style Orange Roughy

1   tablespoon olive oil
5   garlic cloves, coarsely chopped
1   onion, halved and thinly sliced (about 2 cups)
1   green bell pepper, thinly sliced (about 1½ cups)
1   red bell pepper, thinly sliced
1   tomato, chopped (about 1¼ cups)
¾   teaspoon salt
6   (6-ounce) orange roughy fillets
Cooking spray
¼   cup pitted and chopped kalamata olives

Preheat oven to 425°.

Heat oil in a large nonstick skillet over medium-high heat. Add
garlic and next 3 ingredients; sauté 5 to 7 minutes or until vegetables are crisp-tender. Add tomato and salt; cook 2 minutes,
stirring frequently.

Place fish in a 13 x 9-inch baking dish coated with cooking spray.
Place onion mixture on top of fish. Sprinkle with olives. Bake,
uncovered, at 425° for 20 minutes or until fish flakes easily when
tested with a fork. **Yield:** 6 servings.

Per Serving:

Calories 180	**Fiber** 1.5g
Fat 4.9g (sat 0.4g)	**Cholesterol** 34mg
Protein 26.1g	**Sodium** 445mg
Carbohydrate 7.0g	**Exchanges:** 1 Vegetable, 4 Very Lean Meat

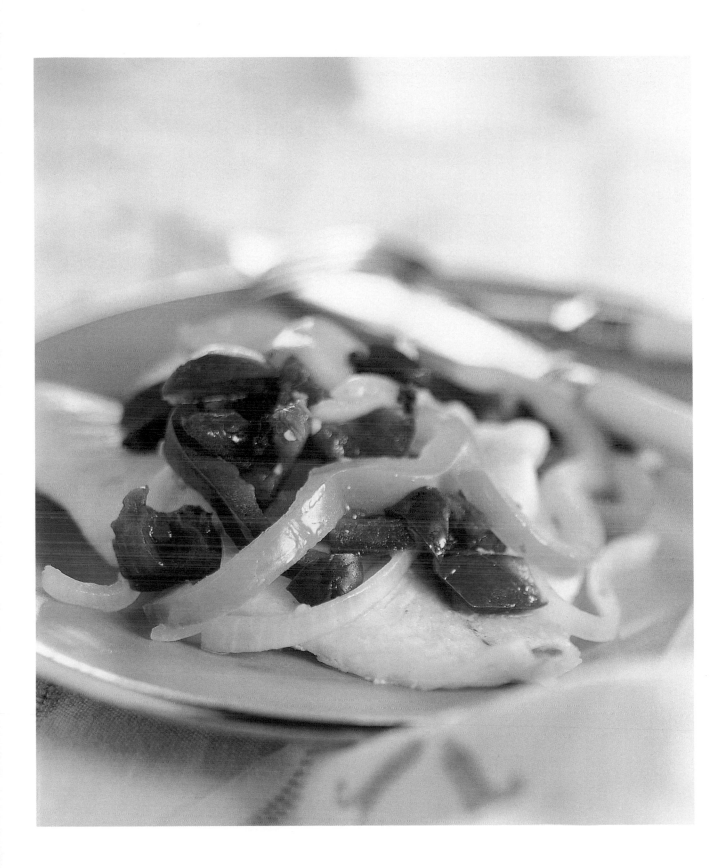

Prep: 11 minutes   Cook: 15 minutes

Lemon-Dill Fish Fillets

½   cup finely crushed plain melba snack crackers (about 20)
1½   teaspoons paprika
1½   teaspoons grated lemon rind
1   teaspoon dried dill
½   teaspoon dry mustard
4   (6-ounce) orange roughy or other lean white fish fillets
Cooking spray
¼   teaspoon salt

Combine first 5 ingredients in a zip-top plastic bag; seal bag, and shake well.

Preheat oven to 400°.

Coat both sides of fish with cooking spray; sprinkle with salt. Place cracker mixture in a shallow dish; dredge fish in cracker mixture. Arrange fish in an 11 x 7-inch baking dish coated with cooking spray. Bake at 400° for 15 minutes or until fish flakes easily when tested with a fork. **Yield:** 4 servings.

Per Serving:

Calories 174	**Fiber** 1.2g
Fat 2.7g (sat 0.1g)	**Cholesterol** 34mg
Protein 27.0g	**Sodium** 367mg
Carbohydrate 9.2g	**Exchanges:** 1 Starch, 3 Very Lean Meat

*super*Quick

Prep: 6 minutes   Cook: 6 minutes

Spicy Lemon Red Snapper

4   (6-ounce) red snapper fillets
¼   cup fresh lemon juice
1   teaspoon black and red pepper blend (such as McCormick's)
1   teaspoon dry mustard
1   teaspoon onion powder
1   teaspoon dried thyme
Cooking spray
Lemon wedges (optional)

Place fish in a large shallow dish; pour lemon juice over fish.
Let stand 5 minutes.

Combine pepper blend and next 3 ingredients. Remove fish from
lemon juice, discarding juice. Rub pepper mixture over both sides
of fillets.

Prepare grill.

Place fish on grill rack or in a grill basket coated with cooking
spray; cover and grill 3 minutes on each side or until fish flakes
easily when tested with a fork. Serve with lemon wedges, if
desired. **Yield:** 4 servings.

Per Serving:

Calories 169	**Fiber** 0.5g
Fat 2.0g (sat 0.4g)	**Cholesterol** 63mg
Protein 33.4g	**Sodium** 91mg
Carbohydrate 2.5g	**Exchanges:** 4 Very Lean Meat

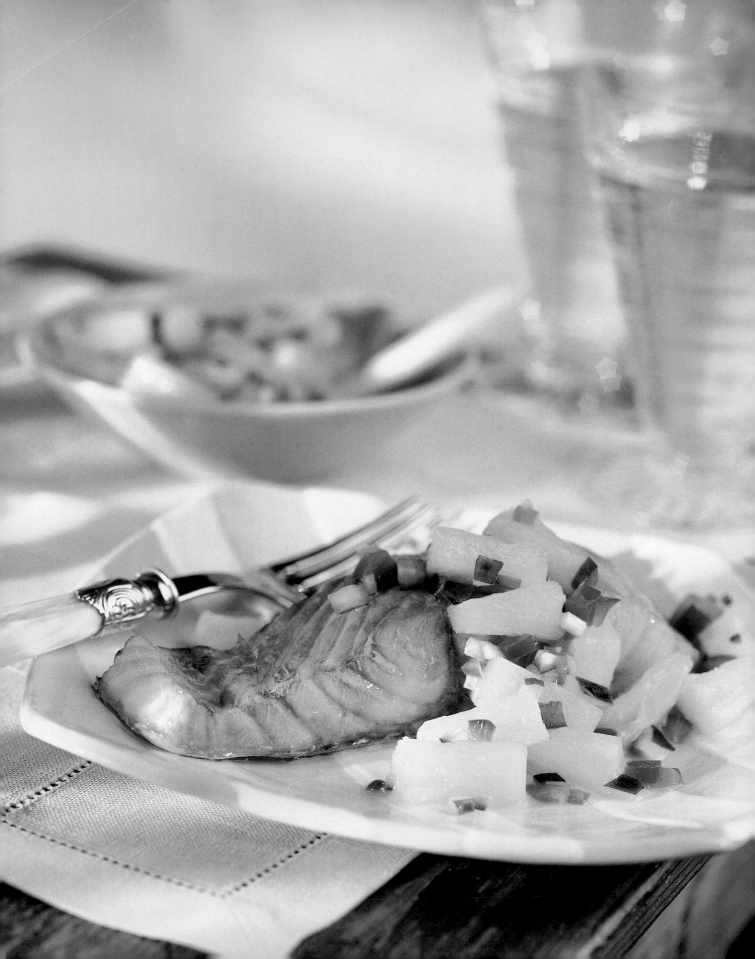

superQuick

Prep: 5 minutes   Cook: 8 minutes

Salmon with Pineapple Salsa

½   cup finely chopped green pepper (about ½ pepper)
¼   cup finely chopped red onion (about ½ small)
1   tablespoon fresh lime juice
1   (20-ounce) can pineapple tidbits in juice, drained
1   jalapeño pepper, seeded and minced
Cooking spray
4   (4-ounce) salmon fillets (about ½ inch thick)
1   tablespoon reduced-sodium soy sauce

Combine first 5 ingredients in a small bowl. Cover and chill.

Preheat broiler.

Arrange fish on rack of a broiler pan coated with cooking spray; brush fish with soy sauce. Broil 4 minutes on each side or until fish flakes easily when tested with a fork. Transfer fish to a serving platter; top evenly with salsa. **Yield:** 4 servings.

Per Serving:

Calories 255
Fat 10.0g (sat 1.7g)
Protein 24.7g
Carbohydrate 15.2g

Fiber 0.5g
Cholesterol 77mg
Sodium 181mg
Exchanges: 1 Fruit, 3 Lean Meat

Use rubber or plastic gloves to protect your skin when handling jalapeños or other hot peppers. To reduce the heat in the salsa, remove the seeds and inner white membranes from the pepper.

Prep: 2 minutes   Marinate: 30 minutes   Cook: 17 minutes

Grilled Salmon with Teriyaki Sauce

¼   cup dry sherry
¼   cup low-sodium soy sauce
1   tablespoon brown sugar
1   tablespoon rice wine vinegar
1   teaspoon garlic powder
½   teaspoon freshly ground black pepper
⅛   teaspoon ground ginger
1   (16-ounce) salmon fillet (about 1 inch thick), skinned
Cooking spray

Combine first 7 ingredients in a shallow dish; stir well. Add fish to dish; cover and marinate in refrigerator 30 minutes.

Prepare grill.

Remove fish from marinade; reserve marinade. Place fish on a grill rack or in a grill basket coated with cooking spray; grill, uncovered, 5 to 7 minutes on each side or until fish flakes easily when tested with a fork. Transfer fish to a serving platter, and keep warm.

Place reserved marinade in a small saucepan; bring to a boil. Boil 5 minutes or until marinade becomes thick and syrupy. Cut fish into 4 equal portions. Spoon evenly over fish, and serve immediately. **Yield:** 4 servings.

Per Serving:

Calories 190	**Fiber** 0.1g
Fat 6.9g (sat 1.3g)	**Cholesterol** 44mg
Protein 25.5g	**Sodium** 548mg
Carbohydrate 4.8g	**Exchanges:** 3½ Lean Meat

Prep: 4 minutes   Cook: 6 minutes

Grilled Tuna with Herbed Mayonnaise

¼   cup fat-free mayonnaise
¼   cup plain fat-free yogurt
1   teaspoon chopped fresh oregano
1   teaspoon chopped fresh tarragon
1   teaspoon lemon juice
¼   teaspoon salt
¼   teaspoon pepper
4   (6-ounce) tuna steaks (about 1 inch thick)
Cooking spray

Combine first 5 ingredients in a small bowl. Cover and chill.

Prepare grill.

Sprinkle salt and pepper over fish. Place fish on grill rack coated with cooking spray; grill 3 minutes on each side or until fish is medium-rare or desired degree of doneness. Top each serving with 2 tablespoons mayonnaise mixture. **Yield:** 4 servings.

Per Serving:

Calories 267	Fiber 0.1g
Fat 8.5g (sat 2.2g)	Cholesterol 65mg
Protein 40.5g	Sodium 414mg
Carbohydrate 4.6g	Exchanges: 5 Lean Meat

Grilled tuna has such great flavor that you may discover your family enjoys eating it more than beef. And it cooks faster, too!

Prep: 10 minutes   Cook: 8 minutes

Tuna with Tapenade

1   tablespoon sun-dried tomato paste
1   (4-ounce) jar capers, drained
1   (4-ounce) jar diced pimiento, drained
15   kalamata olives, pitted
3   garlic cloves, halved
6   (6-ounce) tuna steaks
¼   teaspoon pepper
Cooking spray
Lemon wedges (optional)

Combine first 5 ingredients in a food processor. Pulse 5 times or until finely chopped. Transfer to a bowl, and set aside.

Sprinkle tuna evenly with pepper.

Prepare grill. Place fish on grill rack coated with cooking spray; cover and grill 4 to 6 minutes on each side or until fish flakes easily when tested with a fork. Top each tuna steak with 2 tablespoons olive mixture. Garnish with lemon wedges, if desired. **Yield:** 6 servings.

Per Serving:

Calories 271	**Fiber** 0.3g
Fat 9.8g (sat 2.3g)	**Cholesterol** 65mg
Protein 40.5g	**Sodium** 964mg
Carbohydrate 2.4g	**Exchanges:** 5 Lean Meat

A tapenade is a thick, flavorful paste made from capers and olives. It's also tasty on meat or with low-fat chips or raw vegetables as a dip.

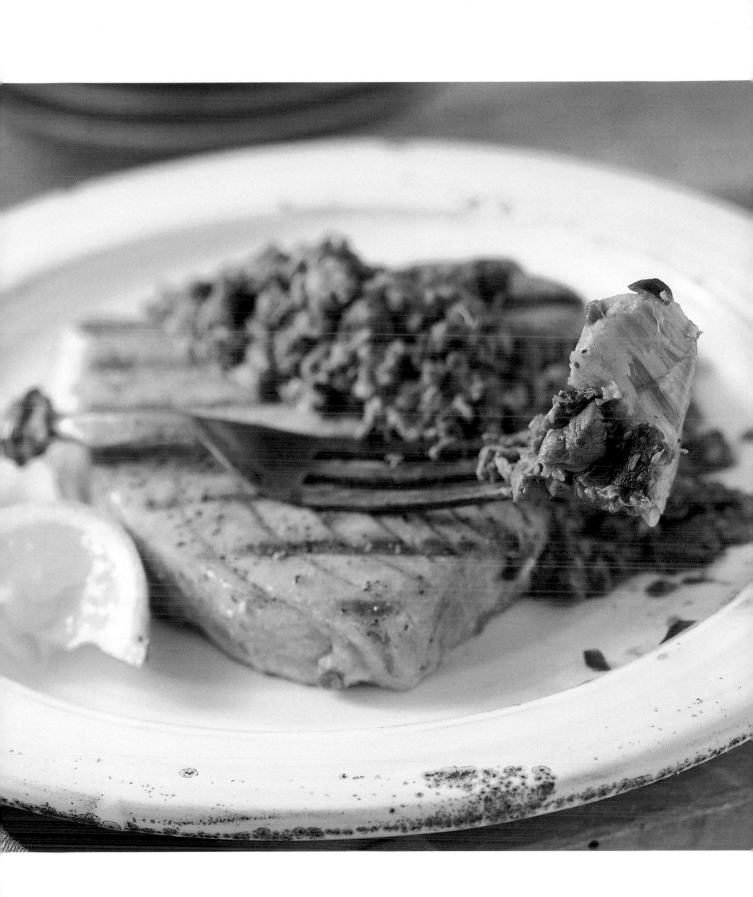

Tuna Casserole

5	ounces uncooked medium egg noodles
1	(10¾-ounce) can condensed reduced-fat, reduced-sodium cream of mushroom soup, undiluted
1	(8.5-ounce) can green peas, drained
1	(6-ounce) can solid white tuna in spring water, drained and flaked
1	(5-ounce) can fat-free evaporated milk
¾	cup (3 ounces) reduced-fat shredded Cheddar cheese
⅓	cup finely chopped onion
½	teaspoon pepper
	Cooking spray
⅔	cup crushed reduced-fat cheese crackers (about 47)

Preheat oven to 350°.

Cook noodles according to package directions, omitting salt and fat; drain. Combine noodles, soup, and next 6 ingredients; pour into an 8-inch square baking dish coated with cooking spray.

Cover and bake at 350° for 30 minutes. Sprinkle with crushed crackers; bake, uncovered, an additional 10 minutes or until thoroughly heated. **Yield:** 4 (1-cup) servings.

Per Serving:

Calories 399	**Fiber** 2.2g
Fat 10.2g (sat 4.6g)	**Cholesterol** 74mg
Protein 29.9g	**Sodium** 916mg
Carbohydrate 46.7g	**Exchanges:** 3 Starch, 3 Lean Meat

This family favorite has been lightened by using reduced-fat soup, fat-free milk, and reduced-fat cheese and crackers.

Prep: 6 minutes   Cook: 9 minutes

Curried Sea Scallops

1   pound sea scallops (about 1 inch thick)
2   teaspoons dark sesame oil
¼   cup orange juice
½   teaspoon curry powder
½   teaspoon freshly ground black pepper
¼   teaspoon salt

Rinse scallops, and pat dry with paper towels. Combine scallops and oil, tossing to coat. Place a large nonstick skillet over high heat until hot. Add half of scallops; cook 2 minutes on each side or until browned. Remove scallops from pan; wipe pan clean with paper towels. Repeat procedure with remaining scallops.

Combine orange juice and next 3 ingredients. Add orange juice mixture to pan. Cook over medium-high heat 1 minute or until thoroughly heated, stirring often. Serve sauce with scallops.
Yield: 4 servings (serving size: about 4 scallops and 2 tablespoons sauce).

Per Serving:

Calories 129	**Fiber** 0.2g
Fat 3.2g (sat 0.4g)	**Cholesterol** 37mg
Protein 19.2g	**Sodium** 328mg
Carbohydrate 4.6g	**Exchanges:** ½ Fruit, 3 Very Lean Meat

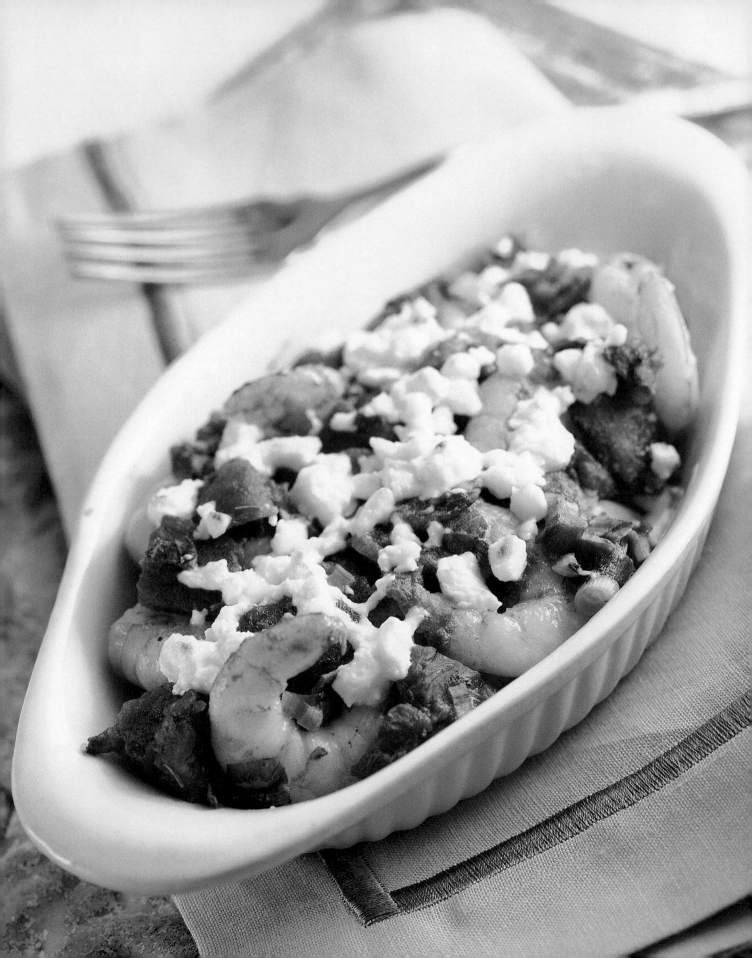

Shrimp with Feta

1	teaspoon olive oil
1	pound peeled and deveined large shrimp
1	cup sliced green onions
4	garlic cloves, minced
1	(14.5-ounce) can diced tomatoes, undrained
1	teaspoon dried oregano
1	teaspoon dried basil
¼	teaspoon sugar
¼	teaspoon ground red pepper
¾	cup (3 ounces) crumbled feta cheese

Preheat broiler.

Heat oil in a large nonstick skillet over medium-high heat. Add shrimp; sauté 3 minutes or until done. Divide shrimp evenly among 4 individual gratin dishes.

Return pan to medium-high heat. Add green onions and garlic; sauté 1 minute. Add tomatoes and next 4 ingredients; cook 3 minutes or until liquid almost evaporates. Spoon tomato mixture evenly over shrimp, and sprinkle with cheese.

Broil 5 minutes or until cheese softens. (Cheese will not melt.) **Yield:** 4 servings.

Per Serving:

Calories 237	**Fiber** 1.5g
Fat 7.6g (sat 3.8g)	**Cholesterol** 282mg
Protein 32.9g	**Sodium** 711mg
Carbohydrate 8.8g	**Exchanges:** 1 Vegetable, 4 Very Lean Meat, ½ Fat

Dilled Shrimp with Angel Hair Pasta

6	ounces uncooked angel hair pasta
2	tablespoons reduced-calorie margarine
¾	cup sliced green onions (about 3 large)
3	tablespoons fresh lemon juice (1 large lemon)
2	large garlic cloves, minced
1	pound peeled and deveined large shrimp
½	cup fat-free half-and-half or fat-free evaporated milk
¼	cup tub-style light cream cheese
2	tablespoons chopped fresh dill or 1½ teaspoons dried dill

Cook pasta according to package directions, omitting salt and fat.

Melt margarine in a large nonstick skillet over medium-high heat. Add green onions, lemon juice, and garlic; sauté 2 minutes. Add shrimp, and cook 5 minutes or until shrimp are done. Remove shrimp from skillet.

Add half-and-half, cream cheese, and dill to pan, stirring until smooth. Cook 1 to 2 minutes or until mixture is bubbly. Return shrimp to pan, and cook until thoroughly heated. Drain pasta; stir in shrimp mixture, and serve immediately. **Yield:** 4 servings (serving size: about 1¼ cups).

Per Serving:

Calories 368	**Fiber** 0.3g
Fat 9.5g (sat 1.8g)	**Cholesterol** 180mg
Protein 31.0g	**Sodium** 366mg
Carbohydrate 37.4g	**Exchanges:** 2½ Starch, 3 Very Lean Meat, 1 Fat

(Photograph on page 61)

Meatless Main

Tomato-Basil Pizza, page 83

Egg Olé Burritos • Southwestern Egg Casserole
Cheese-and-Chile Tortilla Stack • Tomato-Basil Pizza
Mediterranean Pita Rounds • Veggie-Bean Tostadas
Seasoned Cannellini Beans • Meatless Chili
Lentil-Couscous Salad • Broccoli-Tofu Stir-Fry • Spinach Pie

Prep: 11 minutes

Egg Olé Burritos

1	(8-ounce) carton egg substitute
¼	teaspoon salt
¼	teaspoon pepper

Cooking spray

¼	cup (1 ounce) reduced-fat shredded Cheddar cheese
4	(8-inch) flour tortillas
½	cup bottled thick and chunky salsa
¼	cup fat-free sour cream
2	tablespoons chopped fresh cilantro or parsley

Additional bottled salsa (optional)

Combine first 3 ingredients in a small bowl. Coat a large nonstick skillet with cooking spray; place over medium heat until hot. Add egg mixture; cook until mixture is softly set, stirring often. Remove from heat, and top with cheese.

Spoon egg substitute mixture evenly over tortillas; top with salsa, sour cream, and cilantro. Roll up tortillas; place, seam side down, on a serving platter. Serve immediately. Top with additional salsa, if desired. **Yield:** 4 servings.

Per Serving:

Calories 200	**Fiber** 1.6g
Fat 3.6g (sat 0.8g)	**Cholesterol** 5mg
Protein 11.2g	**Sodium** 685mg
Carbohydrate 20.1g	**Exchanges:** 1½ Starch, 1 Lean Meat

Prep: 15 minutes   Chill: 8 hours   Cook: 1 hour, 20 minutes

Southwestern Egg Casserole

12   (6-inch) corn tortillas
8   large eggs
4   large egg whites
2½   cups fat-free milk
1   cup 1% low-fat cottage cheese
¾   teaspoon salt
¾   teaspoon freshly ground black pepper
1½   cups (6 ounces) crumbled feta cheese
1   cup thinly sliced green onions
Cooking spray
1½   cups bottled salsa

Cut tortillas in half; slice tortilla halves crosswise into 1-inch strips.

Combine eggs and egg whites in a large bowl; stir well with a whisk. Stir in milk, cottage cheese, salt, and pepper. Stir in tortilla strips, feta cheese, and onions. Pour into a 13 x 9-inch baking dish coated with cooking spray. Cover and chill 8 hours.

Preheat oven to 325°.

Bake, covered, at 325° for 1 hour. Uncover and bake 20 minutes or just until set (casserole will continue to firm as it cools). Cool 5 minutes, and cut into 12 pieces. Spoon 2 tablespoons salsa over each serving. **Yield:** 12 servings (serving size: 3¼ x 3-inch piece).

Per Serving:

Calories 194   Fiber 1.8g
Fat 7.5g (sat 3.4g)   Cholesterol 156mg
Protein 13.3g   Sodium 517mg
Carbohydrate 18.8g   Exchanges: ½ Starch, 1 Skim Milk, 1 Medium-Fat Meat

Cheese-and-Chile Tortilla Stack

Cooking spray
3   (8-inch) fat-free flour tortillas
1½   cups (6 ounces) preshredded part-skim mozzarella cheese
1   tablespoon plus 1 teaspoon chopped canned jalapeño
         peppers, drained
¾   cup chopped green onions (about 3), divided
2   cups shredded iceberg lettuce
¼   cup fat-free sour cream
¼   cup bottled thick and chunky salsa
2   tablespoons chopped fresh cilantro or parsley

Preheat oven to 400°.

Place 1 tortilla on a baking sheet coated with cooking spray; sprinkle with ¾ cup cheese, 2 teaspoons jalapeño pepper, and ¼ cup green onions. Top with another tortilla, pressing down gently. Sprinkle with remaining cheese, remaining pepper, and ¼ cup green onions. Top with remaining tortilla, pressing down gently. Coat tortilla stack with cooking spray.

Bake at 400° for 6 to 8 minutes or until cheese melts; remove from oven, and transfer to a serving platter. Top with lettuce, sour cream, and salsa. Sprinkle with ¼ cup green onions and cilantro. **Yield:** 3 servings.

Per Serving:

Calories 298	**Fiber** 4.4g
Fat 9.2g (sat 5.8g)	**Cholesterol** 33mg
Protein 20.4g	**Sodium** 603mg
Carbohydrate 32.2g	**Exchanges:** 2 Starch, 2 Medium-Fat Meat

Prep: 5 minutes   Cook: 12 minutes

Tomato-Basil Pizza

1   (10-ounce) Italian cheese-flavored pizza crust (such as Boboli)
⅓   cup pizza sauce
2   ripe tomatoes, thinly sliced
2   teaspoons dried basil or 2 tablespoons chopped fresh basil
¼   cup grated Parmesan cheese
1   cup (4 ounces) preshredded part-skim mozzarella cheese

Preheat oven to 450°.

Place bread shell on a baking sheet; spread with pizza sauce. Top bread shell with tomato slices; sprinkle with basil and Parmesan cheese.

Bake at 450° for 10 minutes. Sprinkle with preshredded cheese; bake 2 to 3 minutes or until crust is golden and cheese melts. Cut into 8 wedges. **Yield:** 4 servings (serving size: 2 wedges).

Per Serving:

Calories 326	**Fiber** 2.5g
Fat 10.9g (sat 4.6g)	**Cholesterol** 22mg
Protein 22.0g	**Sodium** 821mg
Carbohydrate 36.4g	**Exchanges:** 2 Starch, 1 Vegetable, 2 Lean Meat, 1 Fat

(Photograph on page 79)

For a quick meal, serve this pizza with a fruit salad or a piece of fresh fruit.

Prep: 20 minutes   Cook: 11 minutes

Mediterranean Pita Rounds

2   (15-ounce) cans no-salt-added chickpeas (garbanzo beans),
        drained
¼   cup fat-free milk
¼   cup fresh lemon juice
5   garlic cloves
8   (8-inch) pitas
1   teaspoon olive oil
1   (10-ounce) package frozen chopped spinach, thawed, drained,
        and squeezed dry
2   cups chopped tomato
1   cup diced green bell pepper
1   cup diced red bell pepper
½   cup (2 ounces) crumbled feta cheese
⅓   cup sliced ripe olives

Preheat oven to 450°.

Combine first 4 ingredients in food processor; process until smooth,
scraping sides of bowl occasionally.

Arrange pitas on baking sheets; brush with olive oil. Bake at 450°
for 6 minutes. Spread bean mixture evenly over pitas, leaving a
½-inch border. Arrange remaining ingredients evenly over pitas.
Bake at 450° 5 minutes or until thoroughly heated and crust
is crisp. **Yield:** 8 servings.

Per Serving:

Calories 397	**Fiber** 11.9g
Fat 6.6g (sat 1.7g)	**Cholesterol** 6mg
Protein 13.5g	**Sodium** 602mg
Carbohydrate 64.8g	**Exchanges:** 3 Starch, 3 Vegetable, 1 Fat

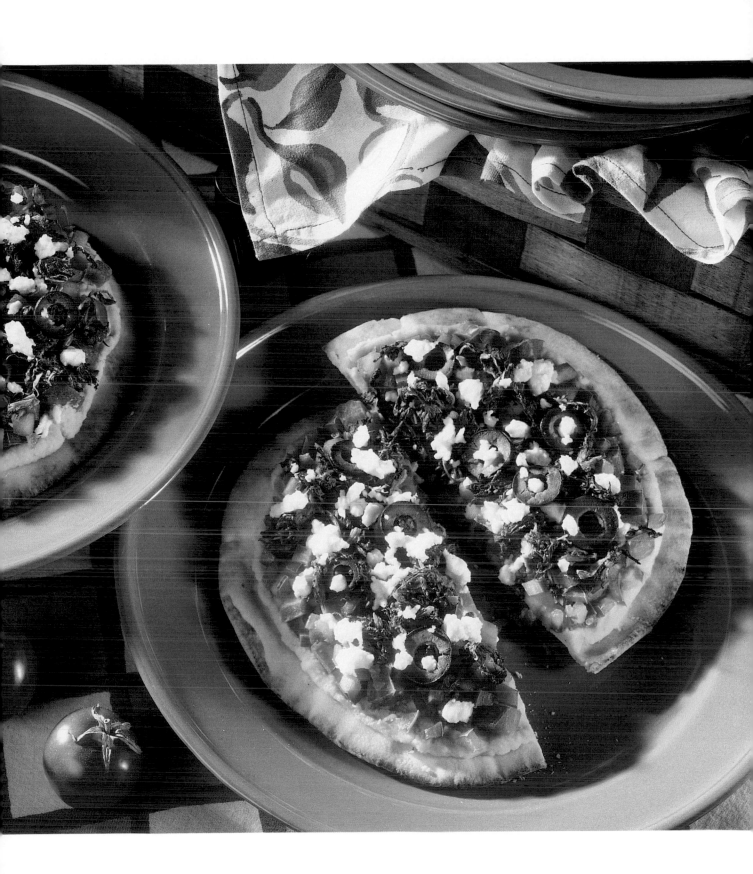

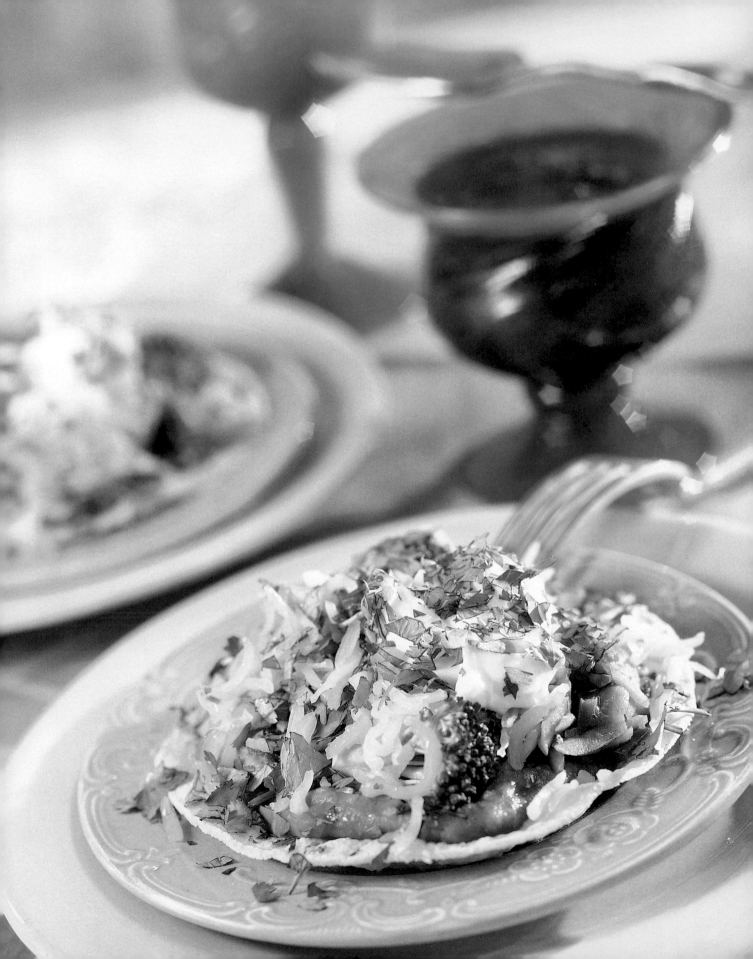

Prep: 18 minutes

Veggie-Bean Tostadas

Cooking spray
1½   cups presliced mushrooms
1½   cups packaged fresh broccoli florets
1   cup packaged shredded carrot
½   cup picante sauce
2   tablespoons water
1   (16-ounce) can fat-free refried beans
4   (6-inch) corn tortillas
1   cup (4 ounces) preshredded reduced-fat Mexican blend or
          Cheddar cheese
1½   tablespoons fat-free sour cream (optional)
¼   cup chopped fresh cilantro (optional)
½   cup picante sauce (optional)

Coat a large nonstick skillet with cooking spray; place over medium-high heat until hot. Add mushrooms and next 4 ingredients; cover and simmer 7 minutes or until vegetables are crisp-tender.

Heat beans according to directions on label.

Preheat broiler. Place tortillas on baking sheet; broil 1 minute on each side or until crisp and golden. Place tortillas on individual serving plates. Top with beans, vegetables, cheese, and, if desired, sour cream, cilantro, and picante sauce. **Yield:** 4 servings.

Per Serving:

Calories 226	Fiber 8.0g
Fat /.1g (sat 4.0g)	Cholesterol 10mg
Protein 16.0g	Sodium 1015mg
Carbohydrate 30.1g	Exchanges: 1 Starch, 2 Vegetable, 2 Lean Meat

Prep: 6 minutes   Cook: 13 minutes

Seasoned Cannellini Beans

1	teaspoon olive oil
2	teaspoons bottled minced garlic
1	cup finely chopped celery
1	cup vegetable broth
2	(15.5-ounce) cans cannellini beans or other white beans, rinsed and drained
1	tablespoon finely chopped fresh sage or 1 teaspoon ground sage
¼	teaspoon salt
¼	teaspoon pepper
¼	cup coarsely chopped fresh flat-leaf parsley
¼	cup (1 ounce) grated fresh Parmesan cheese

Heat oil in a large saucepan over medium-high heat. Add garlic and celery; sauté 3 minutes or until tender. Add broth and next 4 ingredients; bring to a boil. Reduce heat, and simmer, uncovered, 10 minutes.

Spoon beans into individual soup bowls, and sprinkle evenly with parsley and cheese. **Yield:** 4 (1-cup) servings.

Per Serving:

Calories 176	**Fiber** 4.0g
Fat 4.2g (sat 1.7g)	**Cholesterol** 6mg
Protein 10.8g	**Sodium** 821mg
Carbohydrate 22.6g	**Exchanges:** 1½ Starch, 1 Lean Meat

People with Type 2 diabetes may be able to lower their blood glucose levels significantly by eating more soluble fiber, the kind found in beans.

*super*Quick

Prep: 5 minutes   Cook: 13 minutes

Meatless Chili

Cooking spray
2   teaspoons bottled minced garlic
1   large onion, chopped
1   (16-ounce) can chili hot beans, undrained
1   (14.5-ounce) can no-salt-added diced tomatoes, undrained
1   teaspoon chili powder
1   teaspoon ground cumin
12   ounces frozen vegetable and grain protein crumbles (about 3 cups)

Coat a 4-quart saucepan with cooking spray. Place pan over medium-high heat until hot. Add garlic and onion; sauté 3 minutes. Add beans and next 3 ingredients. Bring to a boil, stirring occasionally; reduce heat, and simmer 5 minutes. Add protein crumbles, and cook 3 minutes or until thoroughly heated. **Yield:** 4 (1½-cup) servings.

Per Serving:

Calories 291	**Fiber** 11.4g
Fat 5.9g (sat 0.5g)	**Cholesterol** 0mg
Protein 22.1g	**Sodium** 863mg
Carbohydrate 34.7g	**Exchanges:** 2 Starch, 1 Vegetable, 2 Lean Meat

This chili also works as a burrito filling. Just spoon some chili onto a warm flour tortilla, sprinkle with shredded lettuce and cheese, and roll up the tortilla.

Lentil-Couscous Salad

1   (15-ounce) can lentil and carrot soup (such as Health Valley)
½   cup water
1   (6.1-ounce) package tomato lentil couscous mix
4   cups gourmet salad greens
¼   cup fat-free balsamic vinaigrette
¼   cup (1 ounce) crumbled garlic-flavored feta cheese
¼   cup chopped unsalted peanuts
Apple slices (optional)

Combine soup, water, and seasoning packet from couscous mix in a medium saucepan; bring to a boil. Stir in couscous. Remove from heat; cover and let stand 5 minutes or until liquid is absorbed. Fluff with a fork.

Combine salad greens and vinaigrette; toss gently. Place 1 cup greens on each of 4 plates. Spoon ¾ cup couscous mixture over each serving; sprinkle evenly with crumbled feta cheese and peanuts. Serve with apple slices, if desired (apples not included in analysis). **Yield:** 4 servings.

Per Serving:

Calories 285	**Fiber** 9.0g
Fat 6.5g (sat 1.7g)	**Cholesterol** 6mg
Protein 15.3g	**Sodium** 882mg
Carbohydrate 50.3g	**Exchanges:** 3 Starch, 1 Vegetable, 1 Fat

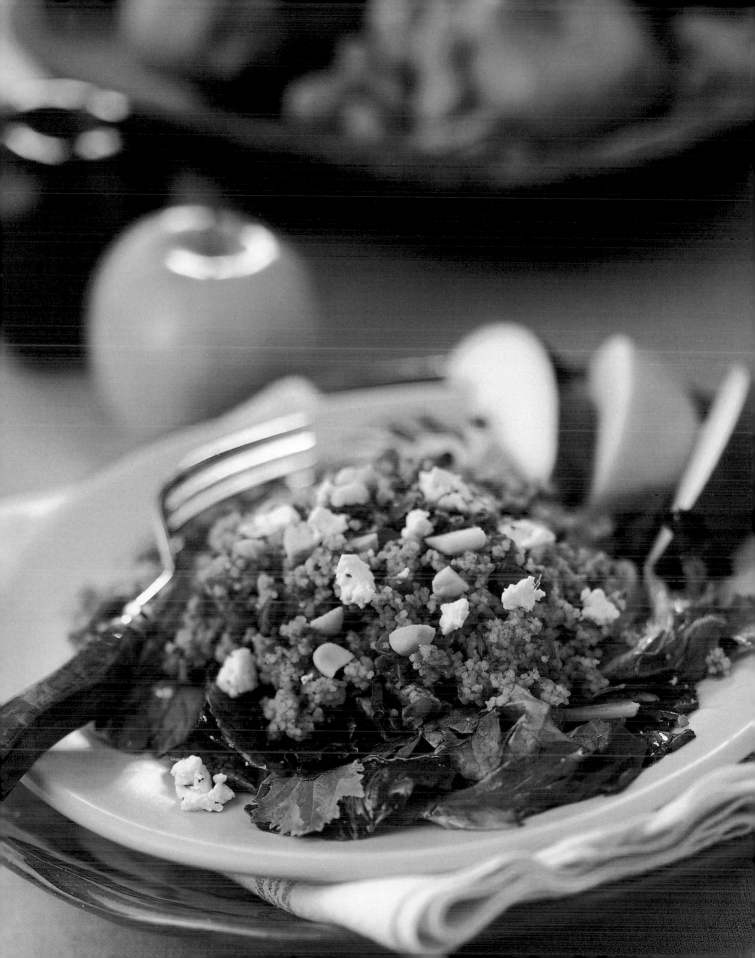

Broccoli-Tofu Stir-Fry

3	tablespoons soy sauce
2	tablespoons rice vinegar
2	teaspoons bottled minced ginger
1½	teaspoons bottled minced garlic
1	(1-pound) package firm tofu, drained and cut into ½-inch cubes
1	tablespoon dark sesame oil, divided
5	cups broccoli florets
½	cup chopped green onions (about 2)
2	tablespoons seeded minced jalapeño pepper
⅓	cup cashews
5	cups hot cooked angel hair pasta (about 11 ounces dry pasta)

Combine first 4 ingredients in a shallow dish. Add tofu, stirring gently to coat. Let stand 15 minutes. Remove tofu from dish, reserving marinade.

Heat 2 teaspoons oil in a nonstick skillet over high heat. Add tofu; cook 2 minutes or until browned. Remove tofu; keep warm.

Add 1 teaspoon oil, broccoli, onions, and jalapeño pepper to pan; sauté 2 minutes. Stir in reserved marinade, tofu, and cashews; cook until thoroughly heated. Serve over pasta. **Yield:** 5 servings (serving size: about 1½ cups stir-fry and 1 cup pasta).

Per Serving:

Calories 358	**Fiber** 5.8g
Fat 11.4g (sat 1.8g)	**Cholesterol** 0mg
Protein 17.5g	**Sodium** 567mg
Carbohydrate 49.0g	**Exchanges:** 2½ Starch, 2 Vegetable, 1 Very Lean Meat, 2 Fat

Let's Talk Tofu

It's Good for You

What is tofu?

Think of tofu as the "cheese" that's made from soy milk. (Soy milk is extracted from ground, cooked soybeans.)

How is it made?

Soy milk curds are drained and pressed in a process similar to cheese making. The firmness of the tofu depends on how much liquid is pressed out.

How does it taste?

Tofu has a bland, slightly nutty flavor, and it takes on the flavor of the food with which it's cooked.

Where do I buy it?

Look for tofu in the fresh produce section of the grocery store or in Asian grocery stores. It's usually either packed in water or vacuum packed. There are several varieties of tofu.
Soft or silken tofu: Use either one of these as a substitute for creamy ingredients in beverages, dips, puddings, soups, and salad dressings.
Firm or extra-firm tofu: Cut it into cubes, slice it, or crumble it; then use it in salads, stir-frys, and pasta dishes.

There are several reasons why you might want to eat tofu:

- Good source of nonmeat protein
- High in calcium, iron, vitamin B, and vitamin E
- Low in saturated fat, cholesterol, and sodium
- Helps increase "good cholesterol" and decrease "bad cholesterol"
- Minimizes symptoms of menopause
- Promotes bone density
- Reduces the risk of certain types of cancer

Hormonelike substances called isoflavones are responsible for most of tofu's health benefits. To get the most from tofu, experts recommend eating 25 to 50 milligrams of isoflavones a day. A half cup of tofu has 40 milligrams of isoflavones. (You can also get isoflavones in other soy products, such as soy milk, miso, and textured soy protein.)

Tofu and Diabetes

There does not appear to be a direct association between tofu and blood glucose, but the potential cholesterol-lowering effect could be important to people with diabetes, who are at higher risk for heart disease.

Spinach Pie

½   cup uncooked long-grain rice
1   cup fat-free, less-sodium chicken broth
1   teaspoon olive oil
1   cup chopped onion (about 1 small)
2   (10-ounce) packages frozen chopped spinach, thawed, drained,
        and squeezed dry
¼   cup (1 ounce) grated fresh Parmesan cheese
1½ cups (6 ounces) preshredded part-skim mozzarella cheese
Cooking spray
2   (8-ounce) packages refrigerated reduced-fat crescent roll dough

Preheat oven to 350°.

Cook rice in chicken broth according to package directions, omitting salt and fat.

Heat oil in a large nonstick skillet over medium heat. Add onion, and sauté 6 minutes or until tender. Combine cooked rice, onion, spinach, and cheeses in a large bowl.

Line bottom and sides of an 11 x 7-inch baking dish coated with cooking spray with 1 package of crescent roll dough. Spoon spinach mixture over dough. Top with remaining package of dough. Bake, uncovered, at 350° for 20 to 25 minutes or until golden. **Yield:** 8 servings (serving size: 2¾ x 1¾-inch piece).

Per Serving:

Calories 360	**Fiber** 2.6g
Fat 14.8g (sat 5.2g)	**Cholesterol** 14mg
Protein 15.1g	**Sodium** 775mg
Carbohydrate 40.8g	**Exchanges:** 2 Starch, 2 Vegetable, 1 High-Fat Meat, 1 Fat

Meats

Steak au Poivre, page 104

Prep: 5 minutes   Cook: 10 minutes

Santa Fe Skillet Casserole

1	pound ground round
¾	cup chopped onion
¾	cup chopped green bell pepper
1½	cups uncooked instant rice (such as Uncle Ben's 5-Minute Rice)
1½	cups low-salt beef broth
¼	teaspoon salt
¼	teaspoon black pepper
1	(14.5-ounce) can Mexican-style stewed tomatoes, undrained
¾	cup (3 ounces) reduced-fat shredded sharp Cheddar cheese

Combine first 3 ingredients in a large nonstick skillet; cook over medium-high heat until beef is browned and vegetables are tender, stirring to crumble beef. (Do not drain.)

Add rice and next 4 ingredients. Cover, reduce heat, and simmer 5 minutes or until rice is tender and liquid is absorbed. Sprinkle with cheese; serve immediately. **Yield:** 6 servings.

Per Serving:

Calories 346	**Fiber** 2.1g
Fat 15.8g (sat 6.8g)	**Cholesterol** 62mg
Protein 21.1g	**Sodium** 488mg
Carbohydrate 28.5g	**Exchanges:** 1½ Starch, 1 Vegetable, 3 Medium-Fat Meat

Your kids will love the taste of this cheesy burger casserole. *You'll* love the fact that you can cook a whole dinner in one pan!

Prep: 10 minutes   Cook: 14 minutes

South-of-the-Border Pizzas

3   (10-inch) flour tortillas
½   pound ground round
1   (15-ounce) can no-salt-added black beans, rinsed and drained
1   (1.25-ounce) package 40%-less-sodium taco seasoning
¼   cup water
2   large tomatoes, finely chopped
½   cup sliced green onions
2   tablespoons chopped fresh cilantro
1   tablespoon minced jalapeño pepper
1   cup preshredded reduced-fat Mexican blend or Cheddar cheese

Preheat oven to 450°. Place tortillas on two baking sheets, and bake at 450° for 2 minutes or until slightly crisp.

Cook beef in a nonstick skillet over medium heat until browned, stirring to crumble. Drain and return to pan. Add beans, taco seasoning, and water; bring to a boil. Reduce heat to low, and simmer 3 minutes, stirring often.

Spread beef mixture over tortillas, leaving a ½-inch border. Combine tomato and next 3 ingredients; sprinkle over beef mixture. Top with cheese.

Bake at 450° for 4 minutes or until tortillas are lightly browned. Remove to a cutting board; let stand 5 minutes. **Yield:** 6 servings (serving size: ½ tortilla with toppings).

Per Serving:

Calories 300	**Fiber** 6.2g
Fat 7.6g (sat 3.2g)	**Cholesterol** 30mg
Protein 21.6g	**Sodium** 641mg
Carbohydrate 40.4g	**Exchanges:** 1½ Starch, 1 Vegetable, 3 Lean Meat

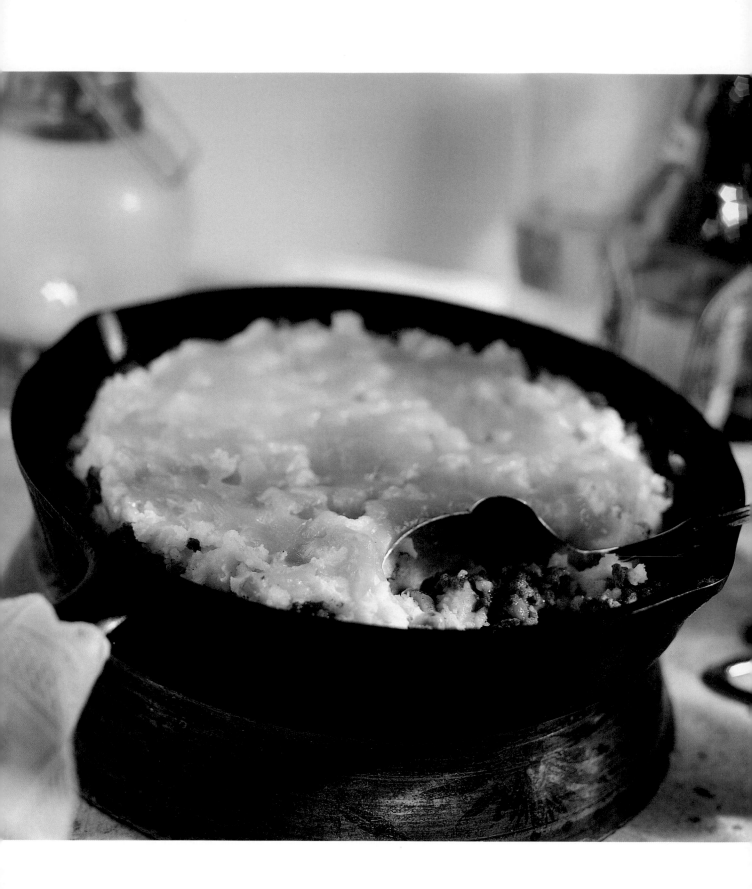

Prep: 8 minutes   Cook: 15 minutes

Speedy Shepherd's Pie

½   (22-ounce) package frozen mashed potatoes (about 3 cups)
1⅓ cups fat-free milk
1   pound ground round
1   cup fresh or frozen chopped onion
1   cup frozen peas and carrots
½   teaspoon pepper
1   (12-ounce) jar fat-free beef gravy
½   cup (2 ounces) reduced-fat shredded Cheddar cheese

Combine potato and milk in a microwave-safe bowl. Microwave at HIGH, uncovered, 8 minutes, stirring once.

Cook beef and onion in a 10-inch ovenproof skillet over medium heat until beef is browned, stirring to crumble. Add peas and carrots, pepper, and gravy. Cook over medium heat 3 minutes or until thoroughly heated, stirring often. Remove from heat.

Spoon potato evenly over beef mixture, leaving a 1-inch border around edge of pan. Broil 3 minutes or until bubbly. Sprinkle with cheese; let stand 5 minutes. **Yield:** 6 servings.

Per Serving:

Calories 236	**Fiber** 1.7g
Fat 6.9g (sat 2.2g)	**Cholesterol** 50mg
Protein 23.4g	**Sodium** 603mg
Carbohydrate 21.8g	**Exchanges:** 1 Starch, 1 Vegetable, 2 Lean Meat

Prep: 5 minutes   Cook: 12 minutes

Spaghetti with Beef, Tomatoes, and Zucchini

1   (7-ounce) package thin spaghetti
½   pound ground round
¼   cup chopped onion
2   (8-ounce) cans no-salt-added tomato sauce
1   teaspoon dried Italian seasoning
½   teaspoon salt
¼   teaspoon garlic powder
¼   teaspoon dried crushed red pepper
1½   cups coarsely chopped zucchini (about 1)
1½   cups coarsely chopped tomato (about 1)

Cook spaghetti according to package directions, omitting salt and fat.

Cook beef and onion in a large nonstick skillet over high heat 4 to 5 minutes or until beef is browned, stirring to crumble. Drain and return to pan. Stir in tomato sauce and next 4 ingredients. Cook over medium heat 2 to 4 minutes or until hot and bubbly, stirring occasionally.

Stir in cooked spaghetti and zucchini. Cook 2 minutes, stirring occasionally. Stir in tomato. **Yield:** 4 (1½-cup) servings.

Per Serving:

Calories 332
Fat 7.9g (sat 2.9g)
Protein 19.3g
Carbohydrate 46.4g
Fiber 2.2g
Cholesterol 35mg
Sodium 336mg
Exchanges: 2 Starch, 2 Vegetable, 2 Lean Meat

Prep: 5 minutes   Marinate: 4 hours   Cook: 8 minutes

Southwestern Grilled Flank Steak

2   tablespoons paprika
1   tablespoon chili powder
2   teaspoons ground cumin
1   teaspoon ground cinnamon
½   teaspoon salt
1   (1½-pound) lean flank steak (about ¾ inch thick)
Cooking spray

Combine first 5 ingredients; rub over both sides of steak. Place steak in a dish; cover and marinate in refrigerator at least 4 hours.

Prepare grill. Place steak on grill rack coated with cooking spray; cover and grill 4 minutes on each side or until desired degree of doneness. Remove steak from grill; let stand 5 minutes before slicing. Cut steak diagonally across the grain into thin slices. **Yield:** 6 servings.

Per Serving:

Calories 271	Fiber 1.1g
Fat 16.5g (sat 6.9g)	Cholesterol 74mg
Protein 27.5g	Sodium 298mg
Carbohydrate 2.6g	Exchanges: 4 Lean Meat, 1 Fat

You'll need to marinate the steak at least 4 hours, but to get even better flavor, let it go overnight.

Beef Fajitas

1   (1-pound) lean flank steak
Cooking spray
½   cup bottled chili sauce
1   tablespoon no-salt-added Creole seasoning
3   cups onion strips
3   cups green, red, and yellow bell pepper strips
6   (8-inch) fat-free flour tortillas
Fresh cilantro sprigs (optional)

Cut steak diagonally across the grain into ¼-inch-thick slices. Coat a large nonstick skillet with cooking spray, and place over medium-high heat until hot. Add steak, chili sauce, and Creole seasoning; cook 4 minutes or until meat is done. Remove from pan. Add onion and bell pepper; sauté 7 minutes or until tender.

Wrap tortillas in wax paper; microwave at HIGH 30 seconds. Spoon steak and vegetable mixture over warm tortillas; wrap or fold tortillas around mixture. Garnish with cilantro sprigs, if desired. **Yield:** 6 servings.

Per Serving:

Calories 317	**Fiber** 3.4g
Fat 9.3g (sat 3.8g)	**Cholesterol** 41mg
Protein 19.7g	**Sodium** 697mg
Carbohydrate 38.6g	**Exchanges:** 2 Starch, 1 Vegetable, 2 Lean Meat

Make your meal a fiesta: serve the fajitas with warm black beans sprinkled with reduced-fat shredded Monterey Jack cheese.

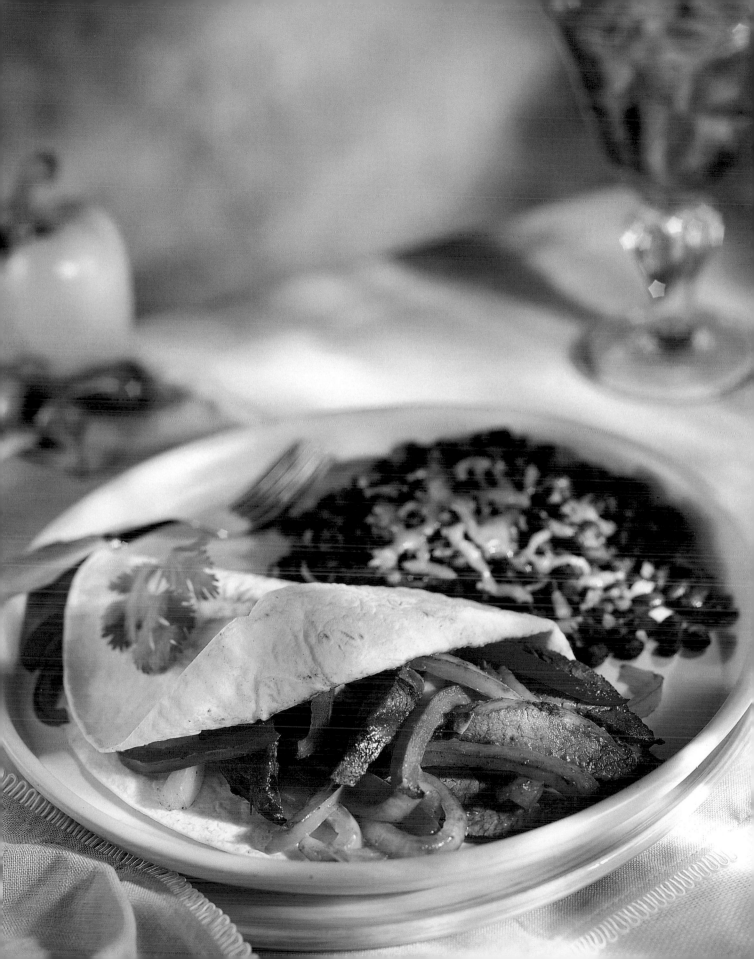

Prep: 1 minute   Cook: 16 minutes

Steak au Poivre

1   tablespoon cracked black pepper
2   (4-ounce) beef tenderloin steaks (1 inch thick)
Cooking spray
¼   cup brandy
½   cup fat-free beef broth
¼   teaspoon salt
¼   teaspoon sugar
3   tablespoons low-fat sour cream

Press cracked black pepper evenly onto both sides of steaks.

Place a large nonstick skillet coated with cooking spray over medium-high heat until hot. Add steaks, and cook 5 minutes on each side or to desired degree of doneness. Transfer to a serving platter; set aside, and keep warm.

Add brandy to pan; let simmer 30 seconds or until liquid is reduced to a glaze. Add beef broth, salt, and sugar. Simmer, uncovered, 4 to 5 minutes or until liquid is reduced by half.

Remove pan from heat; stir in sour cream. Spoon warm sour cream mixture over steaks. **Yield:** 2 servings (serving size: 1 steak and 2 tablespoons sauce).

Per Serving:

Calories 225	**Fiber** 0.8g
Fat 9.0g (sat 3.8g)	**Cholesterol** 75mg
Protein 27.3g	**Sodium** 681mg
Carbohydrate 6.9g	**Exchanges:** ½ Starch, 3½ Lean Meat

(Photograph on page 95)

Prep: 5 minutes   Cook: 8 hours   Stand: 15 minutes

Slow-Cooker Shredded Beef with Chipotle Peppers

1½ pounds top sirloin steak
Cooking spray
1   (16-ounce) package frozen pepper stir-fry
1   (8-ounce) can tomato sauce
¼   cup steak sauce
½   cup chipotle salsa
1   tablespoon sugar
¼   teaspoon salt

Trim fat from steak. Place steak in a 4½-quart electric slow cooker coated with cooking spray. Top with pepper stir-fry. Combine tomato sauce and steak sauce; pour over peppers. Cover with lid; cook on high-heat setting for 1 hour. Reduce heat setting to low; cook 7 hours. Or cover and cook on high-heat setting for 4 hours.

Remove steak from slow cooker with a slotted spoon. Shred steak with 2 forks. Return shredded steak to slow cooker; turn off slow cooker. Add salsa, sugar, and salt. Cover and let stand 15 minutes. **Yield:** 6 servings (serving size: about ¾ cup).

Per Serving:

Calories 272	**Fiber** 1.8g
Fat 9.0g (sat 3.4g)	**Cholesterol** 101mg
Protein 35.0g	**Sodium** 647mg
Carbohydrate 11.5g	**Exchanges:** 2 Vegetable, 3 Lean Meat

Start this recipe in the morning, and you'll have time to go for a walk after work instead of being stuck in the kitchen cooking dinner.

Prep: 5 minutes   Cook: 20 minutes

Beef in Roasted Pepper Gravy

1   (12-ounce) package medium egg noodles
1   (2¼- to 2½-pound) package refrigerated fully cooked beef pot
       roast with gravy
1   (14.5-ounce) can diced tomatoes with onion and garlic, undrained
1   cup frozen small white onions
1   (7-ounce) chopped bottled roasted red bell peppers, drained
½   teaspoon black pepper
½   cup chopped fresh parsley

Cook noodles according to package directions, omitting salt and fat.

Remove pot roast from package, reserving gravy; add gravy to a
4-quart Dutch oven. Add tomatoes, onions, roasted bell pepper,
and black pepper to gravy. Bring gravy mixture to a boil; cover,
reduce heat, and simmer 10 minutes.

Cut pot roast into 2-inch pieces. Add to gravy mixture; cover and
cook 5 minutes.

Drain noodles; toss with parsley. Serve beef mixture over noodles.
Yield: 8 servings (serving size: ¾ cup meat mixture and about
1 cup noodles).

Per Serving:

Calories 391	**Fiber** 1.8g
Fat 8.1g (sat 2.9g)	**Cholesterol** 121mg
Protein 38.2g	**Sodium** 647mg
Carbohydrate 40.1g	**Exchanges:** 2 Starch, 2 Vegetable, 4 Lean Meat

Prep: 10 minutes   Cook: 20 minutes

Italian-Style Veal

4 ounces uncooked vermicelli
¾ pound veal cutlets
½ teaspoon black pepper, divided
2 teaspoons olive oil
2 large red or green bell peppers, cut into strips
¼ cup dry sherry
2 (14.5-ounce) cans diced tomatoes with onion and garlic, undrained
1 teaspoon dried oregano

Cook pasta according to package directions, omitting salt and fat.

Place veal between 2 sheets of heavy-duty plastic wrap, and flatten to ¼-inch thickness using a meat mallet or rolling pin. Cut each cutlet into 2-inch-wide strips; sprinkle with ¼ teaspoon black pepper.

Heat oil in a large nonstick skillet over medium-high heat. Add veal; sauté 2 minutes or until done. Remove veal, using a slotted spoon. Add pepper strips to pan; sauté 5 minutes. Stir in sherry; cook 1 minute. Add tomato, oregano, and ¼ teaspoon black pepper. Bring to a boil; reduce heat, and simmer, uncovered, 5 minutes. Return veal to pan; cook 1 minute or until thoroughly heated.

Drain pasta. To serve, spoon veal mixture over pasta. **Yield:** 4 servings (serving size: 1 cup veal mixture and ½ cup pasta).

Per Serving:

Calories 414
Fat 16.0g (sat 4.9g)
Protein 28.0g
Carbohydrate 41.6g

Fiber 5.0g
Cholesterol 78mg
Sodium 1051mg
Exchanges: 2 Starch, 2 Vegetable, 3 Medium-Fat Meat

Prep: 7 minutes   Cook: 16 minutes

Rosemary-Crusted Lamb Chops

⅓   cup mango chutney
1   tablespoon water
1   tablespoon Dijon mustard
2   teaspoons dried rosemary
8   (4-ounce) lean lamb rib chops, trimmed
½   cup Italian-seasoned breadcrumbs
Cooking spray

Preheat broiler.

Combine first 4 ingredients. Dip chops in chutney mixture; dredge in breadcrumbs.

Place lamb on the rack of a broiler pan coated with cooking spray. Coat tops of lamb chops with cooking spray. Broil 8 minutes. Turn lamb, and broil 6 to 8 minutes or until desired degree of doneness. **Yield:** 4 servings (serving size: 2 chops).

Per Serving:

Calories 238	**Fiber** 1.0g
Fat 8.0g (sat 2.8g)	**Cholesterol** 81mg
Protein 27.4g	**Sodium** 446mg
Carbohydrate 12.9g	**Exchanges:** 1 Starch, 3 Lean Meat

Prep: 10 minutes   Cook: 10 minutes

Oriental Sesame Lamb

1	pound lean boneless lamb, trimmed
1	teaspoon vegetable oil
⅔	cup thinly sliced shallots
1	red bell pepper, cut into thin strips
1	green bell pepper, cut into thin strips
1	large garlic clove, minced
1	tablespoon reduced-sodium soy sauce
1	teaspoon sugar
1	teaspoon rice vinegar
⅛	teaspoon freshly ground black pepper
2	tablespoons sesame seeds, toasted

Slice lamb diagonally across grain into thin strips. Heat oil in a large nonstick skillet over high heat. Add lamb, and stir-fry 2 to 3 minutes or until browned. Remove from pan, and keep warm. Reduce heat to medium-high; add shallots and next 3 ingredients: stir-fry 3 minutes or until crisp-tender.

Return lamb to pan; add soy sauce and next 3 ingredients. Stir-fry until thoroughly heated. Sprinkle with sesame seeds. **Yield:** 5 (1-cup) servings.

Per Serving:

Calories 294	**Fiber** 1.1g
Fat 17.6g (sat 7.1g)	**Cholesterol** 72mg
Protein 19.3g	**Sodium** 180mg
Carbohydrate 8.1g	**Exchanges:** 2 Vegetable, 3 Medium-Fat Meat

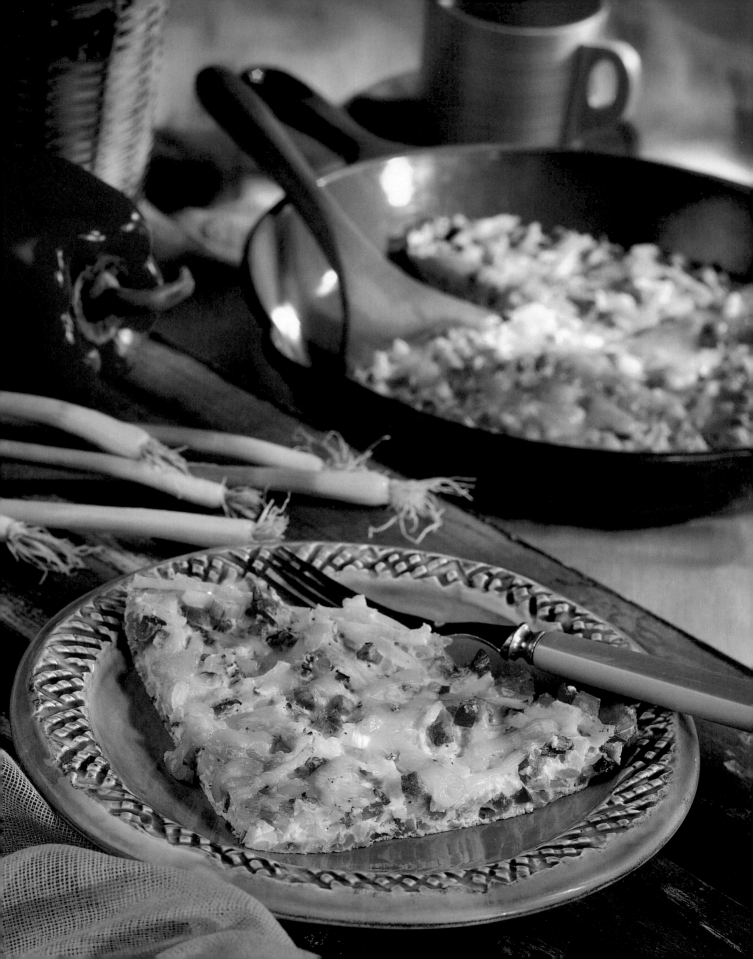

Prep: 10 minutes   Cook: 12 minutes

Ham-and-Potato Frittata

Butter-flavored cooking spray
¾   cup finely chopped reduced-fat, 33%-less-sodium cooked ham
⅓   cup finely chopped red bell pepper (about ½ small)
2   cups frozen country-style hash brown potatoes
½   cup sliced green onions (about 2 large)
¼   teaspoon salt
¼   teaspoon black pepper
1   (8-ounce) carton egg substitute
⅓   cup (1.3 ounces) reduced-fat shredded sharp Cheddar cheese

Preheat oven to 450°. Place a 10-inch nonstick ovenproof skillet coated with cooking spray over medium-high heat until hot. Add ham and bell pepper; sauté 3 minutes. Add potatoes and next 3 ingredients; sauté 4 to 5 minutes or until vegetables are tender.

Reduce heat to medium-low. Add egg substitute; stir gently. Cook 2 to 3 minutes or until nearly set. Place pan in oven, and bake at 450° for 3 to 4 minutes or until set. Sprinkle with cheese while frittata is hot. **Yield:** 4 servings.

Per Serving:

Calories 128	**Fiber** 0.6g
Fat 3.5g (sat 1.6g)	**Cholesterol** 22mg
Protein 14.8g	**Sodium** 550mg
Carbohydrate 9.4g	**Exchanges:** ½ Starch, 2 Lean Meat

A frittata is simply a no-fuss omelet. The basic ingredients are the same, but instead of flipping the egg mixture into a half-moon, you cook the whole recipe in the pan, and cut it into wedges.

super Quick

Prep: 10 minutes   Cook: 10 minutes

Cumin-Rubbed Pork Chops

4   (4-ounce) boneless center-cut loin pork chops
2   teaspoons ground cumin
¼   teaspoon salt
Cooking spray
1   cup diced peeled mango or papaya
1   cup rinsed and drained canned black beans
⅓   cup bottled thick and chunky salsa
¼   cup chopped fresh cilantro or parsley

Prepare grill. Sprinkle both sides of pork with cumin and salt; coat pork with cooking spray. Place pork on grill rack coated with cooking spray; grill, covered, 5 minutes on each side or until done.

Combine mango, beans, and salsa in a small bowl. Serve mango mixture with pork chops; sprinkle with cilantro. **Yield:** 4 servings.

Per Serving:

Calories 315   Fiber 4.0g
Fat 9.6g (sat 3.1g)   Cholesterol 80mg
Protein 32.2g   Sodium 434mg
Carbohydrate 25.7g   Exchanges: 1 Starch, ½ Fruit, 4 Lean Meat

Serve these Southwestern-style chops with warm cornbread sticks and a tossed green salad drizzled with fat-free ranch dressing.

112   Pork

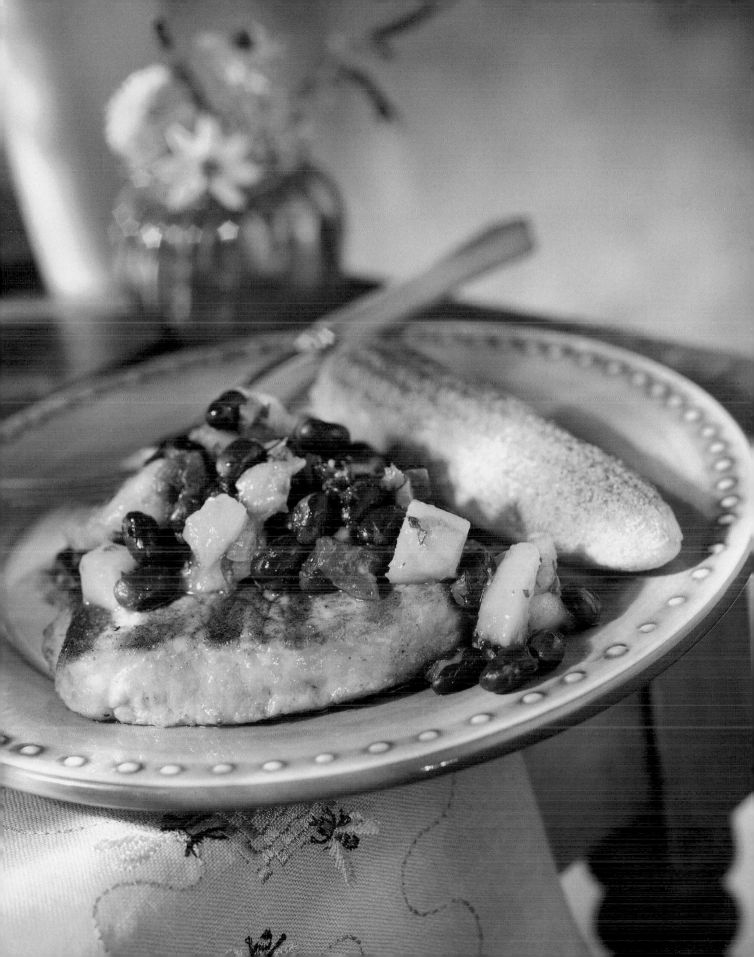

Prep: 5 minutes   Cook: 15 minutes

Pork Medaillons with Pear Sauce

4   (4-ounce) boneless center-cut loin pork chops (about ½ inch thick)
½   teaspoon pepper
¼   teaspoon salt
1   teaspoon margarine
2   firm, ripe pears
1   tablespoon sugar
½   teaspoon dried rosemary, crushed
½   cup apple juice

Sprinkle both sides of pork with pepper and salt. Melt margarine in a large nonstick skillet over medium-high heat. Add pork; cook 3 minutes on each side or until browned. Remove pork from pan; set aside.

Core pears, and cut into ½-inch slices. Add pear slices to pan; sprinkle with sugar and rosemary. Cook over medium-low heat 3 minutes, stirring often.

Pour apple juice into pan; return pork to pan. Simmer 6 to 8 minutes or until pork is done. **Yield:** 4 servings.

Per Serving:

Calories 279	**Fiber** 2.7g
Fat 9.5g (sat 3.0g)	**Cholesterol** 71mg
Protein 25.4g	**Sodium** 234mg
Carbohydrate 23.1g	**Exchanges:** 1½ Fruit, 3 Lean Meat

Poultry

Chicken with Spiced Peach Sauce, page 126

Prep: 5 minutes   Cook: 1 hour

Chicken-Broccoli Casserole

1   cup fat-free mayonnaise
1   tablespoon lemon juice
2   (10¾-ounce) cans condensed reduced-fat, reduced-sodium cream
        of chicken soup, undiluted
Butter-flavored cooking spray
2   (16-ounce) packages frozen broccoli florets
4   cups chopped cooked chicken breast
2   cups (8 ounces) reduced-fat shredded sharp Cheddar cheese
3   (1-ounce) slices white bread, crumbled

Preheat oven to 350°.

Combine first 3 ingredients in a bowl; stir well. Layer broccoli and chicken in a 13 x 9-inch baking dish coated with cooking spray. Top with soup mixture, cheese, and bread. Lightly coat casserole with cooking spray.

Bake, uncovered, at 350° for 1 hour or until bubbly. **Yield:** 10 servings (serving size: about 1½ cups).

Per Serving:

Calories 262	**Fiber** 2.7g
Fat 7.9g (sat 4.2g)	**Cholesterol** 69mg
Protein 29.3g	**Sodium** 699mg
Carbohydrate 20.3g	**Exchanges:** 1 Starch, 1 Vegetable, 3 Lean Meat

For quick chicken, use roasted deli chicken breast (without the skin) or a bag of frozen diced cooked chicken. You'll need about a pound of cooked chicken to get 4 cups of chopped chicken.

Prep: 4 minutes   Cook: 12 minutes

Creamed Chicken over Biscuits

1   (6-ounce) can flaky buttermilk biscuits
Cooking spray
1   (9-ounce) package frozen diced cooked chicken breast
1   teaspoon bottled minced garlic
1   (10-ounce) package frozen mixed vegetables, thawed and drained
¼   cup dry white wine or less-sodium chicken broth
¼   cup water
¼   teaspoon pepper
1   (10¾-ounce) can condensed reduced-fat, reduced-sodium cream
       of roasted chicken with savory herbs soup, undiluted

Preheat oven, and bake biscuits according to package directions.

Coat a large nonstick skillet with cooking spray; place over medium-high heat until hot. Add chicken and garlic; cook 5 minutes, stirring occasionally. Stir in vegetables and remaining 4 ingredients; cook over medium heat 5 minutes or until vegetables are tender and thoroughly heated, stirring often.

Split each biscuit in half, and place on individual serving plates; spoon chicken mixture evenly over biscuits. **Yield:** 5 servings.

Per Serving:

Calories 254	**Fiber** 2.2g
Fat 8.0g (sat 2.2g)	**Cholesterol** 38mg
Protein 17.6g	**Sodium** 718mg
Carbohydrate 28.1g	**Exchanges:** 1½ Starch, 1 Vegetable, 2 Very Lean Meat, 1 Fat

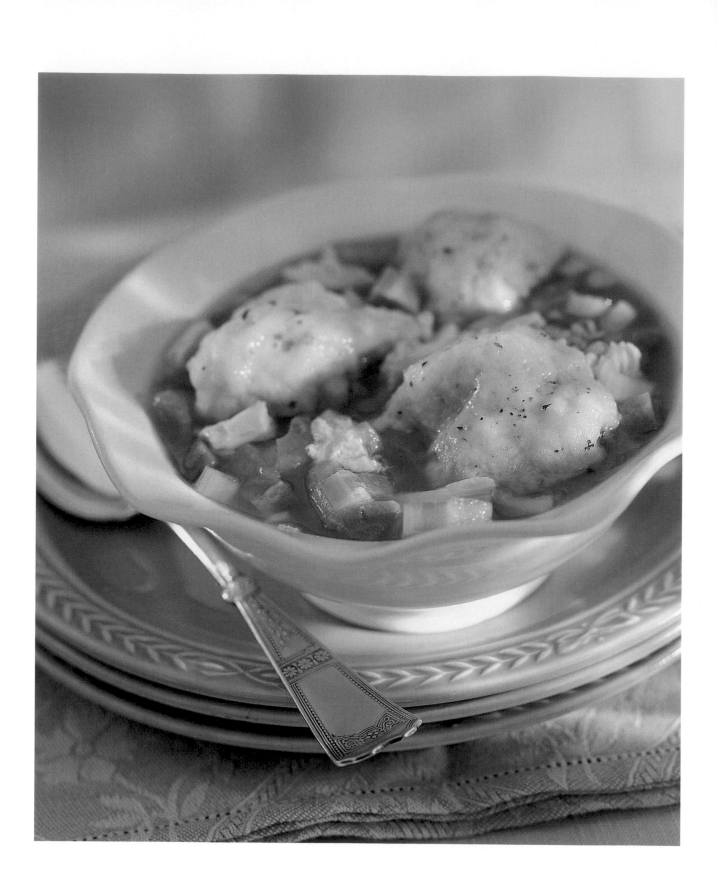

Chicken and Dumplings

1	cup chopped celery (about 3 stalks)
1	cup chopped onion (about 1)
1	cup chopped carrot (about 1)
½	teaspoon salt
¼	teaspoon pepper
4	(14¼-ounce) cans fat-free, less-sodium chicken broth
2	cups low-fat baking mix
1	teaspoon dried parsley flakes
¾	cup fat-free milk
3	cups shredded roasted chicken

Combine first 6 ingredients in a Dutch oven; bring to a boil. Cover, reduce heat to medium, and cook 5 minutes.

Combine baking mix and parsley flakes. Add milk, stirring with a fork just until dry ingredients are moist.

Return broth mixture to a boil. Drop dough by teaspoonfuls into boiling broth; reduce heat to medium. Cover and cook 10 minutes, stirring once.

Add chicken to broth mixture, stirring gently. Cook, uncovered, 5 minutes or until thoroughly heated. **Yield:** 6 servings.

Per Serving:

Calories 330	**Fiber** 1.4g
Fat 9.2g (sat 2.1g)	**Cholesterol** 54mg
Protein 24.1g	**Sodium** 636mg
Carbohydrate 34.4g	**Exchanges:** 2 Starch, 1 Vegetable, 2 Medium-Fat Meat

Cook: 10 minutes

Szechuan Chicken and Vegetables

2	teaspoons dark or light sesame oil
1	pound chicken breast tenders
¼	teaspoon dried red pepper flakes
1	(10-ounce) package fresh stir-fry vegetables (about 2½ cups)
¼	cup low-sodium teriyaki sauce

Heat oil in a large nonstick skillet over medium-high heat. Add chicken, and sprinkle with pepper flakes; stir-fry 3 minutes.

Add vegetables and teriyaki sauce; stir-fry 5 minutes or until vegetables are crisp-tender and chicken is thoroughly cooked. Serve over noodles, if desired (noodles not included in analysis). **Yield:** 4 servings.

Per Serving:

Calories 183	**Fiber** 1.2g
Fat 3.7g (sat 0.7g)	**Cholesterol** 66mg
Protein 28.8g	**Sodium** 341mg
Carbohydrate 7.9g	**Exchanges:** 2 Vegetable, 3 Very Lean Meat

If you want to serve the chicken and vegetables with noodles, boil water first so the noodles can cook while you're stir-frying.

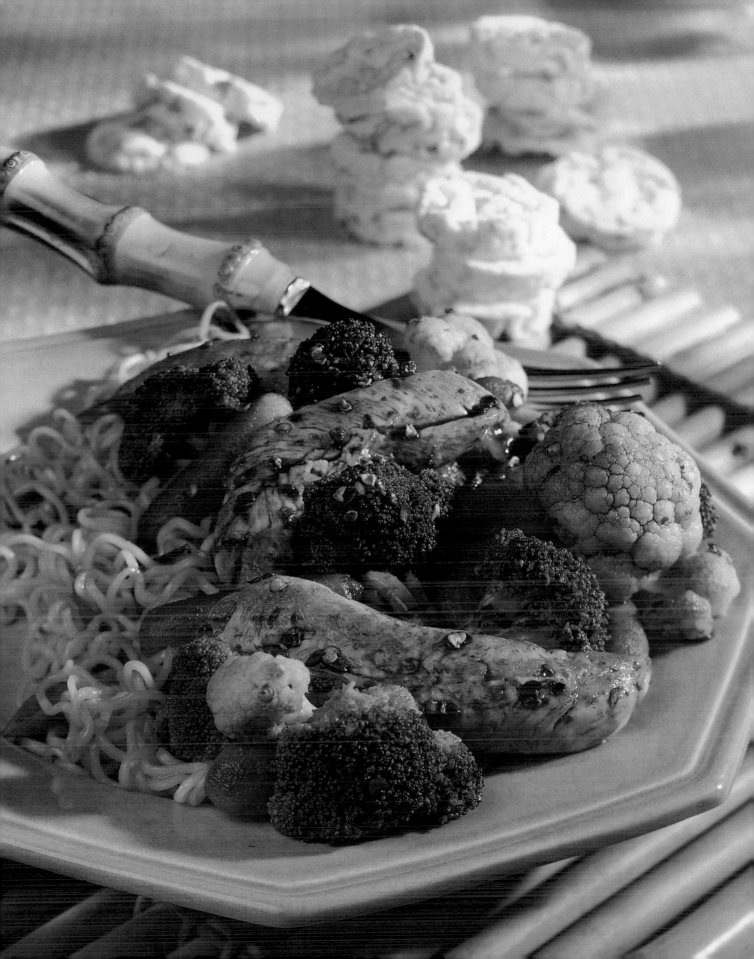

superQuick

Prep: 3 minutes   Cook: 12 minutes

Curry-Orange Chicken

2   cups uncooked instant rice
¾   pound chicken breast tenders
2   tablespoons all-purpose flour
Cooking spray
1   teaspoon vegetable oil
2   green bell peppers, cut into strips
1   tablespoon bottled minced garlic
½   cup fat-free, less-sodium chicken broth
⅓   cup low-sugar orange marmalade
1   teaspoon curry powder

Cook rice according to package directions, omitting salt and fat.

Combine chicken and flour in a zip-top plastic bag. Seal bag, and shake gently to coat chicken.

Coat a nonstick skillet with cooking spray; add oil. Place over medium-high heat until hot. Add pepper strips and garlic; sauté 1 minute. Add chicken, and sauté 6 minutes or until chicken is lightly browned. Add broth, marmalade, and curry powder; cook 5 minutes or until chicken is done, stirring often. Serve over rice.
Yield: 4 servings.

Per Serving:

Calories 323	Fiber 1.7g
Fat 3.1g (sat 0.6g)	Cholesterol 49mg
Protein 24.6g	Sodium 81mg
Carbohydrate 47.1g	Exchanges: 3 Starch, 2 Very Lean Meat

Prep: 5 minutes   Cook: 11 minutes

Creole Chicken Pasta

3	tablespoons all-purpose flour
2	teaspoons no-salt-added Creole seasoning, divided
4	(4-ounce) skinless, boneless chicken breast halves, cut into strips
2	teaspoons hot pepper oil
1	onion, cut into vertical strips (about 1 cup)
1	green pepper, cut into julienne strips
1	teaspoon bottled minced garlic
1	(9-ounce) package refrigerated fettuccine
1	cup fat-free half-and-half or fat-free evaporated milk

Combine flour and 1½ teaspoons Creole seasoning in a large heavy-duty zip-top plastic bag; add chicken, and shake to coat.

Heat oil in a large nonstick skillet over medium-high heat. Add chicken, onion, pepper, and garlic; cook 8 to 10 minutes or until chicken is done and vegetables are tender, stirring occasionally.

Cook fettuccine according to package directions, omitting salt and fat; drain well.

Combine ½ teaspoon Creole seasoning and half-and-half; add to chicken mixture in pan, scraping pan to loosen browned bits. Cook 1 minute or until sauce thickens slightly. Toss with cooked pasta; serve immediately. **Yield:** 6 (1-cup) servings.

Per Serving:

Calories 269	**Fiber** 2.0g
Fat 3.7g (sat 0.5g)	**Cholesterol** 44mg
Protein 23.4g	**Sodium** 172mg
Carbohydrate 32.2g	**Exchanges:** 2 Starch, 3 Very Lean Meat

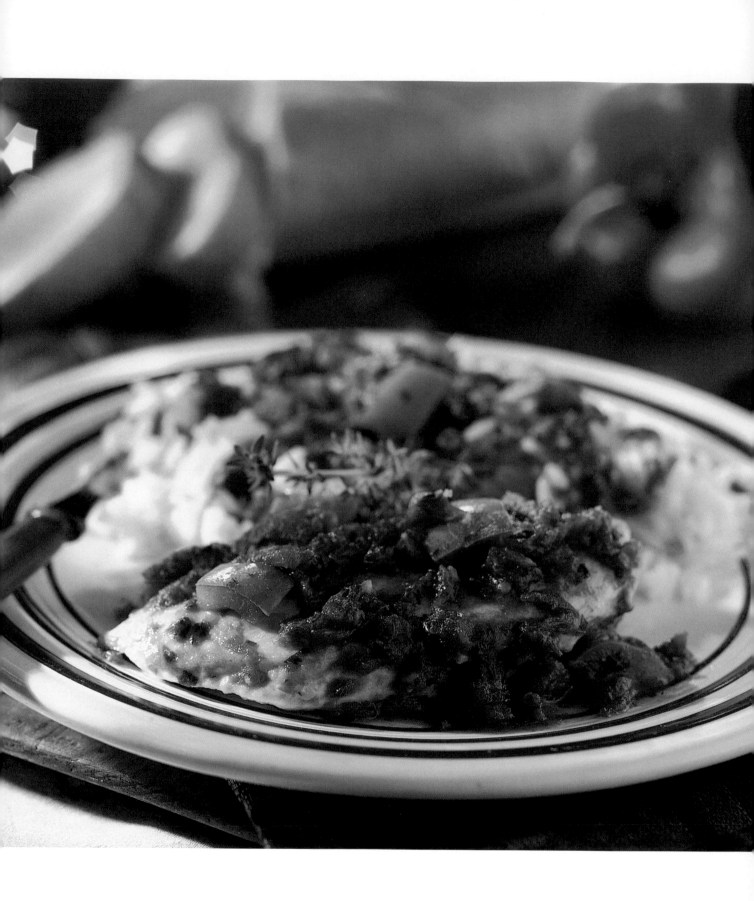

Prep: 5 minutes   Cook: 19 minutes

Cajun Fire Chicken

Cooking spray
2   teaspoons olive oil
4   (4-ounce) skinless, boneless chicken breast halves
1   green bell pepper, coarsely chopped
1   (14½-ounce) can stewed tomatoes, undrained and chopped
2   teaspoons hot sauce
⅓   cup chopped fresh cilantro, divided
½   teaspoon dried thyme
Additional hot sauce (optional)
Fresh thyme sprigs (optional)

Heat oil in a large nonstick skillet coated with cooking spray over medium-high heat. Add chicken, and cook 2 minutes on each side or until lightly browned. Add pepper, tomatoes, 2 teaspoons hot sauce, ¼ cup cilantro, and dried thyme. Bring to a boil; cover, reduce heat, and simmer 5 minutes. Uncover and simmer 10 minutes.

Stir remaining cilantro into tomato mixture. Serve with additional hot sauce, and garnish with thyme sprigs, if desired. **Yield:** 4 servings.

Per Serving:

Calories 192	**Fiber** 2.1g
Fat 3.8g (sat 0.7g)	**Cholesterol** 66mg
Protein 27.6g	**Sodium** 323mg
Carbohydrate 11.8g	**Exchanges:** 2 Vegetable, 3 Very Lean Meat

Steam quick-cooking rice in the microwave to serve with this saucy dish.

Chicken with Spiced Peach Sauce

1   (16-ounce) can sliced peaches in light syrup, undrained
¼   cup low-sugar orange marmalade
¼   teaspoon salt
¼   teaspoon ground nutmeg
¼   teaspoon ground ginger
⅛   teaspoon pepper
Cooking spray
6   (4-ounce) skinless, boneless chicken breast halves
1   teaspoon cornstarch
2   tablespoons water

Drain peaches, reserving ½ cup syrup. Set peaches aside. Combine ½ cup syrup, marmalade, and next 4 ingredients.

Place a large nonstick skillet coated with cooking spray over medium-high heat until hot. Add chicken, and cook 5 minutes or until browned on both sides, turning once. Add peaches and marmalade mixture to chicken; bring to a boil. Cover and cook 10 minutes or until chicken is done. Remove chicken from pan, and keep warm.

Combine cornstarch and water; add to peach mixture. Bring to a boil; cook, stirring constantly, 1 minute or until sauce thickens. Spoon sauce evenly over chicken. **Yield:** 6 servings.

Per Serving:

Calories 165	**Fiber** 0.6g
Fat 1.6g (sat 0.4g)	**Cholesterol** 66mg
Protein 26.8g	**Sodium** 178mg
Carbohydrate 8.4g	**Exchanges:** 1 Fruit, 3 Very Lean Meat

(Photograph on page 115)

Prep: 2 minutes   Cook: 17 minutes

Raspberry-Glazed Chicken

Butter-flavored cooking spray
4   (4-ounce) skinless, boneless chicken breast halves
¼   teaspoon salt
¼   teaspoon pepper
¼   cup raspberry spread (such as Polaner All Fruit), divided
1   teaspoon water

Place chicken on the rack of a broiler pan or roasting pan coated with cooking spray. Sprinkle salt and pepper evenly over chicken. Broil 7 minutes. Turn chicken; baste with 2 tablespoons raspberry spread, and broil 10 minutes or until chicken is done.

Combine 2 tablespoons raspberry spread and 1 teaspoon water in a 1-cup glass measure. Microwave at HIGH 30 seconds; spoon mixture evenly over chicken. **Yield:** 4 servings.

Per Serving:

Calories 167	Fiber 0.0g
Fat 3.1g (sat 0.8g)	Cholesterol 70mg
Protein 25.8g	Sodium 224mg
Carbohydrate 7.5g	Exchanges: ½ Fruit, 3 Very Lean Meat

For a simple flavor variation, use low-sugar orange marmalade or peach spread.

Prep: 5 minutes   Marinate: 8 hours   Cook: 10 minutes

Tropical Grilled Chicken

¾ teaspoon Jamaican jerk seasoning (such as Spice Islands)
4 (4-ounce) skinless, boneless chicken breast halves
1 cup canned light coconut milk
½ cup orange juice
1 tablespoon minced fresh basil
¼ teaspoon salt
Cooking spray
2 teaspoons flour

Rub jerk seasoning on chicken. Combine coconut milk and next 3 ingredients in a small bowl. Pour half of mixture into a large heavy-duty zip-top plastic bag; add chicken. Seal bag, and marinate in refrigerator at least 8 hours. Cover and store remaining coconut milk mixture in refrigerator.

Prepare grill. Remove chicken from marinade, discarding marinade. Place chicken on grill rack coated with cooking spray; grill, covered, 5 minutes on each side or until done.

Pour reserved coconut milk mixture into a small saucepan; add flour. Place over medium-high heat. Bring to a boil; reduce heat, and simmer, uncovered, 5 minutes or until slightly thick. Serve sauce over chicken. **Yield:** 4 servings.

Per Serving:

Calories 179	**Fiber** 0.1g
Fat 5.4g (sat 2.2g)	**Cholesterol** 70mg
Protein 26.6g	**Sodium** 184mg
Carbohydrate 5.3g	**Exchanges:** 3 Lean Meat

Thai Chicken and Plums

1   tablespoon salt-free Thai seasoning (such as The Spice Hunter)
¼   teaspoon pepper
⅛   teaspoon salt
6   (3-ounce) skinless, boneless chicken thighs, quartered
1   teaspoon vegetable oil
4   plums, pitted and quartered
¼   cup fat-free, less-sodium chicken broth
¼   cup low-sugar apricot or peach preserves
1   tablespoon red wine vinegar

Combine first 3 ingredients in a heavy-duty zip-top plastic bag, and add chicken. Seal bag; shake chicken to coat.

Heat oil in a large nonstick skillet over medium-high heat. Add chicken; cook 6 minutes, turning to brown all sides. Remove chicken from pan.

Add plums to pan, scraping pan to loosen browned bits. Cook 1 minute on each side or until skins are browned. Add chicken broth to pan. Stir in apricot preserves and red wine vinegar; stir well. Return chicken to pan. Bring to a boil; cover, reduce heat, and simmer 5 minutes or until chicken is done. **Yield:** 4 servings.

Per Serving:

Calories 237	**Fiber** 1.2g
Fat 6.6g (sat 1.5g)	**Cholesterol** 106mg
Protein 25.8g	**Sodium** 232mg
Carbohydrate 18.2g	**Exchanges:** 1 Fruit, 3 Lean Meat

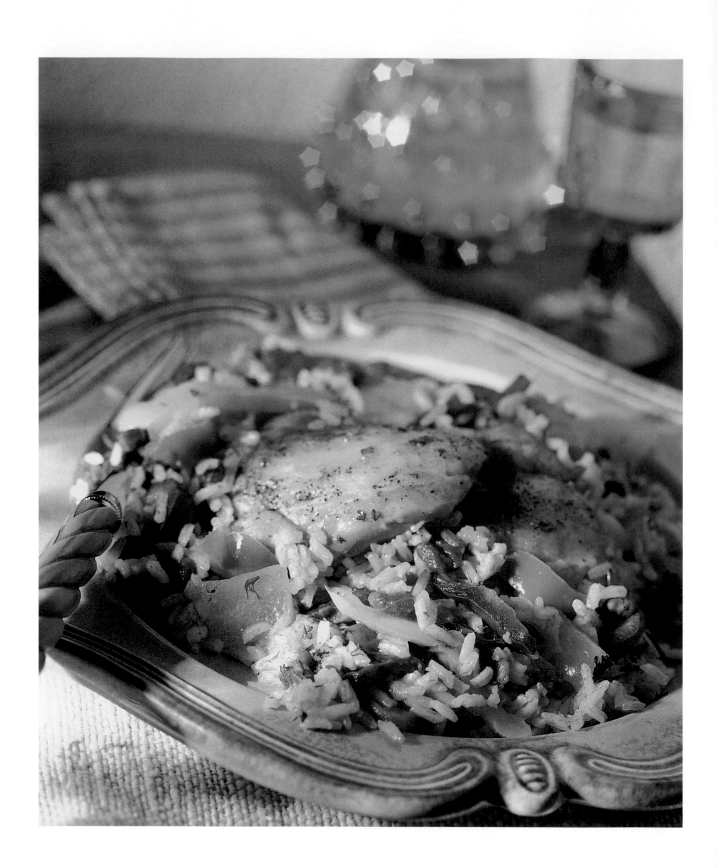

Spanish-Style Chicken

1	tablespoon olive oil
1	pound skinless, boneless chicken thighs
½	teaspoon salt
½	teaspoon pepper
1	(16-ounce) package frozen pepper stir-fry (such as Birds Eye)
1	(14½-ounce) can diced tomatoes, undrained
1	cup uncooked long-grain rice
1	cup water
½	cup dry sherry
½	teaspoon dried rosemary
2	tablespoons drained capers
2	tablespoons minced fresh parsley

Heat oil in a Dutch oven over medium-high heat. Sprinkle chicken with salt and pepper; add chicken to pan. Cook 6 minutes, turning to brown all sides.

Add pepper stir-fry and next 5 ingredients; stir well. Bring to a boil; cover, reduce heat, and simmer 22 minutes or until liquid is almost absorbed. Stir in capers and parsley. Cover and let stand 5 minutes. **Yield:** 4 servings.

Per Serving:

Calories 353	**Fiber** 3.3g
Fat 7.6g (sat 1.5g)	**Cholesterol** 82mg
Protein 24.4g	**Sodium** 738mg
Carbohydrate 44.3g	**Exchanges:** 2½ Starch, 1½ Vegetable, 2 Lean Meat

Prep: 5 minutes   Cook: 1 ½ hours

Teriyaki Roast Chicken

1   (3-pound) roasting chicken
1   small onion, quartered
⅓   cup low-sodium teriyaki sauce
1   teaspoon garlic-pepper seasoning
Cooking spray

Preheat oven to 375°.

Remove giblets from chicken. Reserve for another use. Rinse and drain chicken; pat dry.

Place onion in cavity of chicken. Brush chicken on all sides with some of the teriyaki sauce. Sprinkle with garlic-pepper seasoning. Place chicken, breast side up, on a rack in a roasting pan coated with cooking spray. Insert meat thermometer into meaty part of thigh, making sure it does not touch the bone. Pour remaining teriyaki sauce over chicken.

Bake, uncovered, at 375° for 1½ hours or until meat thermometer registers 185°. Remove skin before serving. **Yield:** 6 servings.

Per Serving:

Calories 170	**Fiber** 0.4g
Fat 6.1g (sat 1.6g)	**Cholesterol** 73mg
Protein 24.3g	**Sodium** 271mg
Carbohydrate 3.0g	**Exchanges:** 1 Vegetable, 3 Lean Meat

Serve this peppery chicken with orange rice:
Start with boil-in-bag rice; stir in a dash of salt and
grated orange rind. Garnish with orange slices.

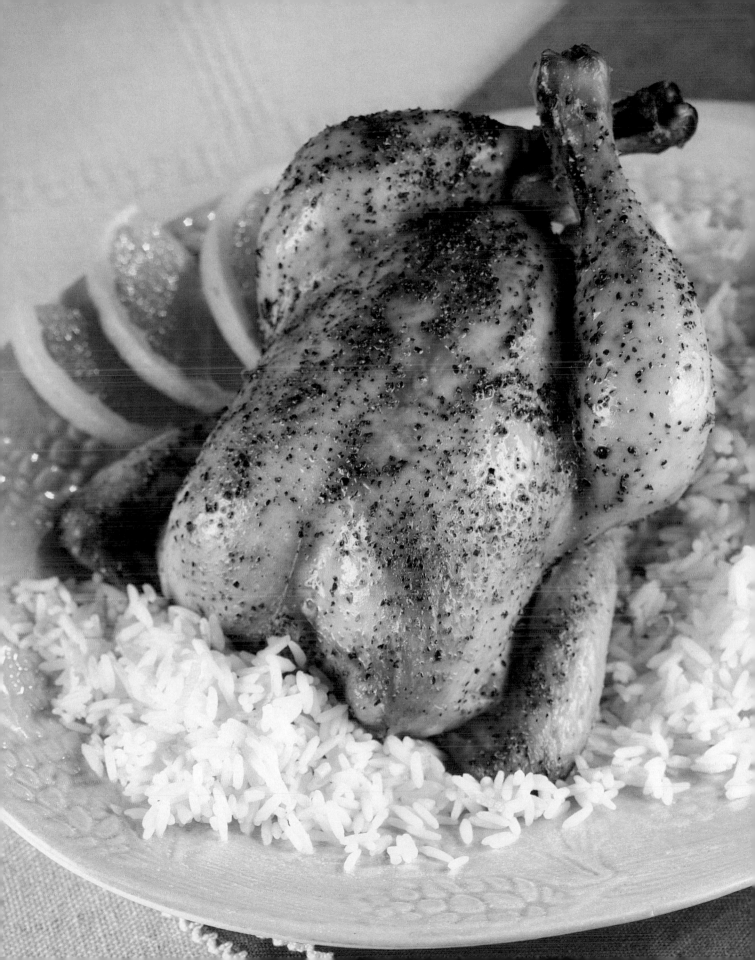

Prep: 5 minutes   Cook: 12 minutes

Turkey Pepperoni Pizza

1   (10-ounce) Italian cheese-flavored pizza crust (such as Boboli)
½   cup pizza sauce
2   ounces turkey pepperoni
1   red or green bell pepper, seeded and cut into thin slices
1   cup (4 ounces) preshredded part-skim mozzarella cheese

Preheat oven to 450°.

Place pizza crust on a baking sheet. Spread pizza sauce over crust; top with pepperoni and pepper slices. Bake at 450° for 10 minutes.

Sprinkle cheese over pizza; bake 2 minutes or until cheese melts. Cut into wedges. **Yield:** 6 servings (serving size: 1 wedge).

Per Serving:

Calories 216	**Fiber** 1.1g
Fat 7.7g (sat 3.3g)	**Cholesterol** 29mg
Protein 14.0g	**Sodium** 604mg
Carbohydrate 22.3g	**Exchanges:** 1½ Starch, 1½ Medium-Fat Meat

An easy pizza deserves an easy salad, so open a bag of fat-free Caesar salad mix. And while you're opening packages, have a no added sugar ice cream bar for dessert.

Prep: 5 minutes   Cook: 15 minutes

Spicy Turkey Skillet

1	(15-ounce) can no-salt-added black beans, drained
1	(10-ounce) can diced tomatoes and green chiles, undrained
1	(8¾-ounce) can no-salt-added whole-kernel corn, drained
2	tablespoons chopped fresh cilantro or parsley
1	teaspoon ground cumin
½	teaspoon hot sauce

Cooking spray

1	pound turkey breast tenderloin, cut into 1-inch pieces
¾	cup chopped onion
½	teaspoon bottled minced garlic

Combine first 6 ingredients in a bowl.

Place a large nonstick skillet coated with cooking spray over medium-high heat until hot. Add turkey, onion, and garlic; cook until turkey is browned, stirring to crumble. Stir in bean mixture; bring to a boil. Reduce heat, and simmer, uncovered, 5 to 7 minutes or until turkey is done and most of liquid is evaporated, stirring occasionally. **Yield:** 4 servings.

Per Serving:

Calories 288	**Fiber** 8.7g
Fat 2.6g (sat 0.6g)	**Cholesterol** 68mg
Protein 35.2g	**Sodium** 327mg
Carbohydrate 28.7g	**Exchanges:** 1½ Starch, 1 Vegetable, 4 Very Lean Meat

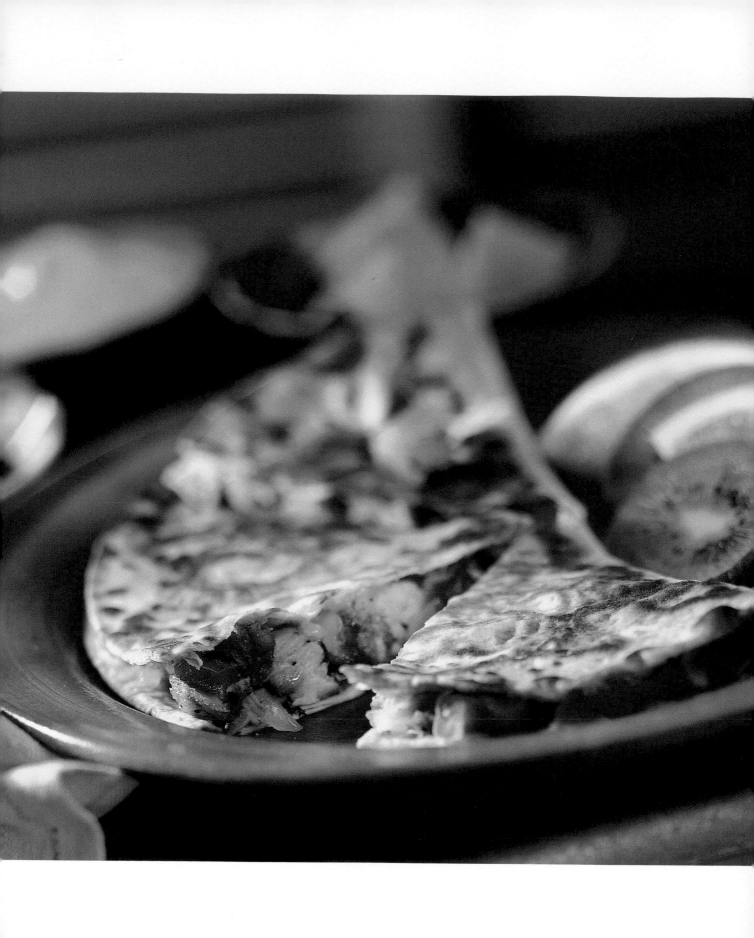

Turkey Quesadillas

½   teaspoon vegetable oil
¾   cup chopped green bell pepper (about 1 small)
½   cup chopped red onion (about 1 small)
1   teaspoon ground cumin
1   cup chopped cooked turkey breast
¾   cup drained no-salt-added diced tomatoes
½   cup minced fresh cilantro
½   teaspoon salt
⅛   teaspoon freshly ground black pepper
4   (8-inch) fat-free flour tortillas
⅓   cup (1.5 ounces) shredded reduced-fat Monterey Jack cheese
Cooking spray

Heat oil in a large nonstick skillet over medium-high heat. Add chopped pepper and onion; sauté 3 minutes. Add cumin; sauté 1 minute. Add turkey and tomato; sauté 3 minutes. Stir in cilantro, salt, and black pepper.

Place about ½ cup turkey mixture on half of each tortilla. Sprinkle cheese evenly over turkey; fold tortillas in half. Coat a large nonstick skillet with cooking spray; place over medium-high heat until hot. Add 2 filled tortillas; cook 30 seconds on each side or until lightly browned. Set aside, and keep warm. Repeat procedure with remaining 2 tortillas. Cut each folded tortilla into 3 wedges. **Yield:** 4 servings (serving size: 3 wedges).

Per Serving:

Calories 205	**Fiber** 2.3g
Fat 3.5g (sat 1.5g)	**Cholesterol** 20mg
Protein 12.5g	**Sodium** 648mg
Carbohydrate 29.8g	**Exchanges:** 2 Starch, 1 Lean Meat

Prep: 5 minutes   Cook: 11 minutes

Turkey with Tarragon-Mustard Cream

Cooking spray
1   pound turkey cutlets
½   cup fat-free milk
1   tablespoon all-purpose flour
⅓   cup reduced-fat sour cream
2   teaspoons Dijon mustard
1½ teaspoons chopped fresh or ½ teaspoon dried tarragon
½   teaspoon sugar
Dash of salt

Place a large nonstick skillet coated with cooking spray over medium-high heat until hot. Add turkey; cook 2 minutes on each side or until browned. Set turkey aside, and keep warm.

Combine milk and flour in a small bowl, stirring well with a whisk. Place milk mixture in a small saucepan; bring to a boil over medium heat, stirring often. Remove from heat; stir in sour cream and remaining 4 ingredients. Cook over low heat just until heated, stirring often. (Do not boil.) Serve sauce over turkey cutlets.
Yield: 4 servings.

Per Serving:

Calories 233	**Fiber** 0.1g
Fat 10.8g (sat 3.8g)	**Cholesterol** 85mg
Protein 27.2g	**Sodium** 195mg
Carbohydrate 5.2g	**Exchanges:** 4 Lean Meat

Salads

Steak Caesar Salad for Two, page 160

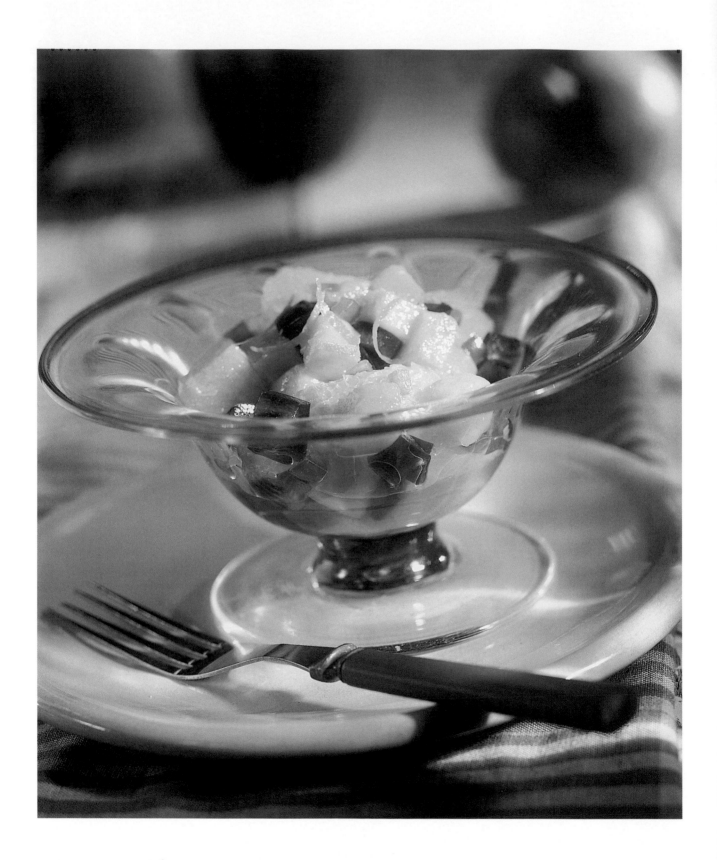

Prep: 15 minutes   Stand: 10 minutes

Pineapple-Mango Salad

1 cup fresh pineapple chunks
¾ cup cubed peeled ripe mango (about 1)
¾ cup chopped red bell pepper (about 1)
1 orange
2 tablespoons finely chopped seeded jalapeño pepper (about 1)
1½ tablespoons sugar

Combine first 3 ingredients in a medium bowl; set aside.

Grate 1 teaspoon rind from orange. Peel orange, and cut out sections over a small bowl; squeeze membranes to extract juice. Reserve 2 tablespoons juice. Discard remaining juice and membranes. Add reserved orange rind and sections to mango mixture. Add jalapeño pepper, reserved orange juice, and sugar; toss gently. Let stand 10 minutes. **Yield:** 5 (½-cup) servings.

Per Serving:

Calories 77	**Fiber** 2.0g
Fat 0.2g (sat 0.1g)	**Cholesterol** 0mg
Protein 0.6g	**Sodium** 2mg
Carbohydrate 19.2g	**Exchanges:** 1½ Fruit

Be sure to wear plastic gloves when handling fresh jalapeños so that your skin won't get burned.

Pineapple-Orange Congealed Salad

1   (20-ounce) can crushed pineapple in juice, undrained
1   (0.6-ounce) package sugar-free orange-flavored gelatin
2   cups low-fat buttermilk
1   (12-ounce) container frozen reduced-calorie whipped topping,
        thawed
½   cup chopped pecans

Place pineapple in a small saucepan; cook over medium heat until thoroughly heated. Add gelatin, stirring until gelatin dissolves. Let cool.

Stir in buttermilk. Gently fold in whipped topping and pecans. Pour into a 13 x 9-inch baking dish. Cover and chill 2 to 3 hours or until firm. **Yield:** 16 servings (serving size: 3¼ x 2¼-inch piece).

Per Serving:

Calories 118	**Fiber** 0.6g
Fat 5.7g (sat 3.1g)	**Cholesterol** 2mg
Protein 2.2g	**Sodium** 56mg
Carbohydrate 13.4g	**Exchanges:** 1 Starch, 1 Fat

*super*Quick

Prep: 5 minutes

Red-and-Green Salad

3   cups mixed salad greens
½   cup sweetened dried cranberries (such as Craisins)
¼   cup walnut pieces
3   sliced green onions
⅓   cup fat-free raspberry vinaigrette

Combine first 4 ingredients in a medium bowl. Pour raspberry vinaigrette over salad mixture, and toss well. **Yield:** 4 (¾-cup) servings.

Per Serving:

Calories 112	Fiber 2.3g
Fat 4.5g (sat 0.0g)	Cholesterol 0mg
Protein 2.8g	Sodium 125mg
Carbohydrate 21.1g	Exchanges: 1 Fruit, 1 Vegetable, 1 Fat

This colorful salad works well as an accompaniment to holiday entrées. If you need to make some last-minute substitutions, use raisins instead of cranberries and pecans instead of walnuts.

super Quick

Prep: 6 minutes

Salad Greens with Grapes and Blue Cheese

6   cups torn Bibb lettuce (about 1 head)
1   cup seedless red grapes
2   tablespoons chopped pecans, toasted
2   tablespoons crumbled blue cheese
¼   cup fat-free raspberry vinaigrette

Combine first 4 ingredients; toss with vinaigrette. **Yield:** 4 (1½-cup) servings.

Per Serving:

Calories 97	**Fiber** 1.6g
Fat 4.3g (sat 1.1g)	**Cholesterol** 3mg
Protein 2.6g	**Sodium** 81mg
Carbohydrate 13.7g	**Exchanges:** 1 Fruit, 1 Fat

Red grapes, especially the skins, are rich in compounds called phytonutrients, which may reduce the risk of heart disease and cancer.

Prep: 5 minutes

Italian-Style Salad

1	(10-ounce) bag Italian salad greens (about 6 cups)
½	cup roasted red pepper in water, drained and chopped
2	tablespoons grated fresh Parmesan cheese
⅓	cup fat-free Italian salad dressing

Combine salad greens and roasted red pepper in a large bowl. Sprinkle with Parmesan cheese. Drizzle with dressing, and toss well. **Yield:** 6 (1-cup) servings.

Per Serving:

Calories 25	**Fiber** 1.0g
Fat 0.6g (sat 0.3g)	**Cholesterol** 1mg
Protein 1.6g	**Sodium** 279mg
Carbohydrate 3.7g	**Exchange:** 1 Vegetable

When buying bagged salads, select varieties such as Italian greens that have a lot of dark leaves in the mix. The darker the greens, the more nutrients they contain.

Prep: 20 minutes

Greek Salad Bowl

1   (14-ounce) can quartered artichoke hearts, drained
1   cup sliced cucumber
⅓   cup crumbled feta cheese
12   kalamata olives
1   large tomato, cut into thin wedges
⅓   cup fresh lemon juice
1   tablespoon olive oil
½   teaspoon dried oregano
½   teaspoon lemon pepper seasoning
1   garlic clove, crushed
Freshly ground black pepper (optional)

Combine first 5 ingredients in a large bowl. Combine lemon juice and next 4 ingredients in a small bowl; stir with a whisk until blended. Pour over vegetable mixture; toss to coat. Sprinkle with pepper, if desired. **Yield:** 6 (¾-cup) servings.

Per Serving:

Calories 97	Fiber 2.0g
Fat 5.9g (sat 1.3g)	Cholesterol 6mg
Protein 3.1g	Sodium 236mg
Carbohydrate 10.2g	Exchanges: 2 Vegetable, 1 Fat

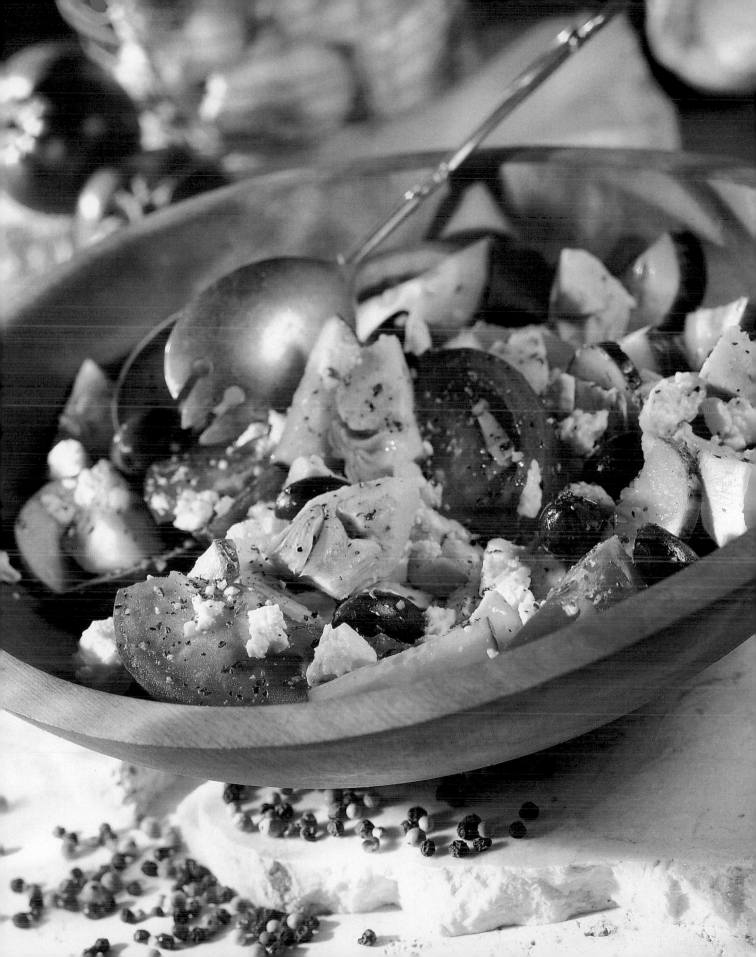

superQuick

Prep: 9 minutes

Cherry Tomato-Cucumber Salad

¼ cup plain fat-free yogurt
2 tablespoons crumbled feta cheese
¼ teaspoon salt
Dash of pepper
1 small garlic clove, crushed
1½ cups cherry tomatoes, halved
1 cucumber, quartered lengthwise and sliced crosswise
(about 1½ cups)

Combine first 5 ingredients in a medium bowl. Add tomato and cucumber; toss gently. Serve immediately. **Yield:** 4 (¾-cup) servings.

Per Serving:

Calories 44	**Fiber** 1.4g
Fat 1.4g (sat 0.8g)	**Cholesterol** 5mg
Protein 2.5g	**Sodium** 222mg
Carbohydrate 6.1g	**Exchange:** 1 Vegetable

super Quick

Prep: 10 minutes

Broccoli-Tomato Salad

2   cups chopped red leaf lettuce
1   cup small broccoli florets
½   cup chickpeas (garbanzo beans)
1   small tomato, cut into wedges
¼   cup fat-free red wine vinaigrette

Combine first 4 ingredients in a medium bowl. Add vinaigrette, and toss well. **Yield:** 5 (1-cup) servings.

Per Serving:

Calories 52	**Fiber** 2.2g
Fat 0.6g (sat 0.0g)	**Cholesterol** 0mg
Protein 1.8g	**Sodium** 189mg
Carbohydrate 10.7g	**Exchanges:** 2 Vegetable

Broccoli is in the cruciferous family of vegetables. Other family members include bok choy, cabbage, collards, and turnips. This clan fights cancer and protects against strokes.

Prep: 5 minutes   Cook: 5 minutes

Wild Rice Salad with Peas

1   (6.2-ounce) package fast-cooking recipe long-grain and wild rice
        (such as Uncle Ben's)
1   (10-ounce) package frozen green peas, thawed
⅔   cup chopped red bell pepper
½   cup sliced almonds, toasted
⅓   cup teriyaki sauce

Cook rice mix according to package directions, omitting seasoning packet and fat.

Combine rice mix, peas, bell pepper, almonds, and teriyaki sauce in a large bowl. Stir well, and let cool. Serve at room temperature. **Yield:** 6 (1-cup) servings.

Per Serving:

Calories 203	**Fiber** 3.6g
Fat 4.6g (sat 0.5g)	**Cholesterol** 0mg
Protein 7.1g	**Sodium** 616mg
Carbohydrate 33.7g	**Exchanges:** 2 Starch, 1 Fat

The Fiber Factor

Health benefits of fiber

What is fiber?

Fiber is the part of plant foods that your body cannot digest. It's a vital component of food that promotes good health.

There are two kinds of fiber: **insoluble** and **soluble**. Insoluble fiber does not dissolve in water, and soluble fiber does. Insoluble fiber is known as roughage and is found in such foods as whole grain breads and cereals, most vegetables, and the skins of fruits and root vegetables. Soluble fiber dissolves and becomes gummy in water. It's found in dried peas and beans, oats, barley, psyllium seed husks, apples, oranges, and carrots.

How does fiber affect diabetes?

For some people with diabetes, soluble fiber helps control blood sugars and may reduce the need for insulin or other diabetes medications. Because the fiber slows the time for the stomach to empty, it takes longer for the glucose to get into the blood.

To increase your soluble fiber, add at least two servings a day of dried peas or beans, oats, apples, or oranges as part of your total fiber intake.

How much do I need?

The health experts say that 20 to 35 grams of total fiber (soluble and insoluble) each day may help lower fasting blood glucose levels in some people with diabetes. On average, people in the United States eat about 11 grams of fiber per day.

- Helps prevent constipation
- Decreases risk of diverticulosis
- Reduces chance of hemorrhoids
- Reduces risk of colon cancer
- Reduces risk of rectal cancer
- Helps control blood glucose in people with diabetes
- Helps lower cholesterol
- Reduces risk of heart disease
- Aids in weight loss

Note: If you are over 65 years of age and have had surgery of any part of your stomach, intestines, or colon, check with your doctor before adding fiber to your diet.

151

make *Ahead*

Prep: 14 minutes   Chill: 8 hours

Bean and Pasta Salad

8   ounces uncooked farfalle (bow tie pasta)
1   (15-ounce) can no-salt-added black beans, rinsed and drained
1   pint cherry tomatoes, halved
1   green bell pepper, chopped
1   large lime, cut in half
2   tablespoons chopped fresh cilantro
2   garlic cloves, minced
1   cup fat-free Italian dressing
3   tablespoons grated fresh Parmesan cheese

Cook pasta according to package directions, omitting salt and fat.

Place beans, tomatoes, and pepper in a large bowl. Squeeze lime juice over bean mixture; discard lime rind. Add cilantro and garlic to bean mixture.

Drain pasta; add to bean mixture. Pour dressing over salad, tossing gently to coat; sprinkle with cheese. Cover and chill at least 8 hours. **Yield:** 6 (1½-cup) servings.

Per Serving:

Calories 276	**Fiber** 3.5g
Fat 2.3g (sat 0.7g)	**Cholesterol** 2mg
Protein 12.3g	**Sodium** 659mg
Carbohydrate 51.6g	**Exchanges:** 3 Starch, 1 Vegetable, 1 Very Lean Meat

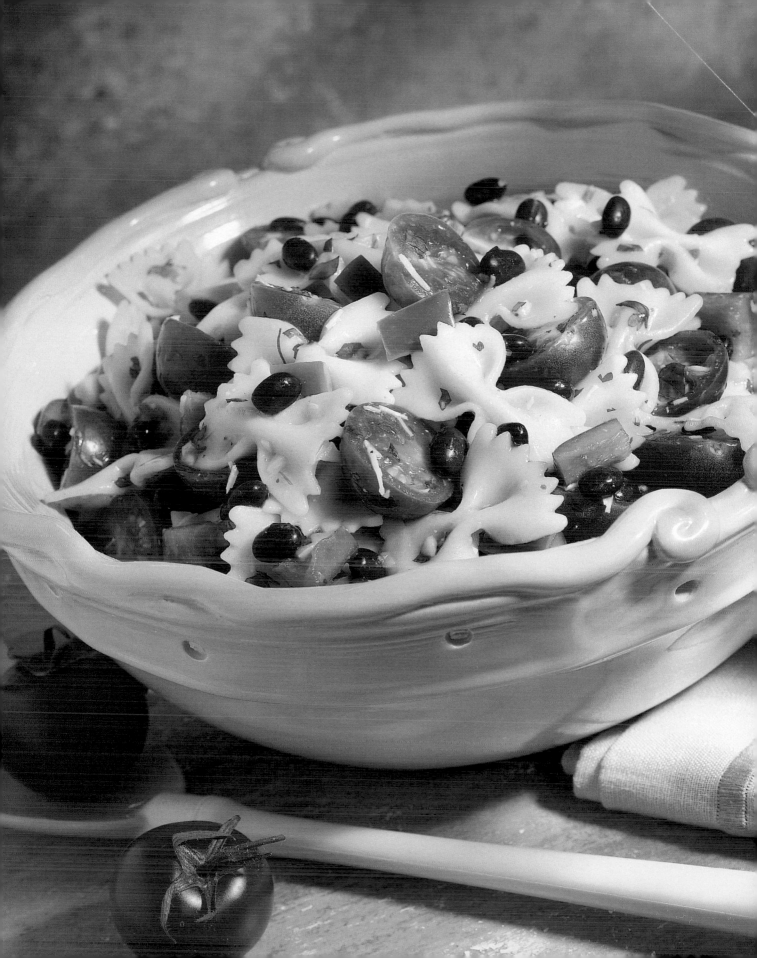

Prep: 8 minutes   Cook: 8 minutes

Fruited Chef's Salad with Garlic Croutons

4   ounces French bread, cut into 12 slices
Garlic-flavored cooking spray
2   tablespoons chopped walnuts
8   cups packed mixed salad greens
1   ripe pear, cored and diced (about 1¼ cup)
4   ounces reduced-sodium deli ham, cut into thin strips
¼   cup crumbled blue cheese
⅓   cup fat-free raspberry vinaigrette

Preheat oven to 400°.

Spray both sides of bread slices with cooking spray. Arrange bread on a large baking sheet, and bake at 400° for 4 minutes. Turn bread; add walnuts to pan, and bake 4 additional minutes or until croutons are golden.

Arrange salad greens on 4 salad plates. Arrange pear, ham, and cheese over greens. Drizzle vinaigrette evenly over salads, and sprinkle with toasted walnuts. Serve with toasted croutons.
Yield: 4 servings.

Per Serving:

Calories 203	**Fiber** 2.7g
Fat 6.4g (sat 1.7g)	**Cholesterol** 20mg
Protein 11.1g	**Sodium** 638mg
Carbohydrate 26.8g	**Exchanges:** 1 Starch, ½ Fruit, 1 Vegetable, 1 Lean Meat

Prep: 5 minutes   Cook: 3 minutes   Chill: 1 hour

Coleslaw with Shrimp

4   cups water
8   ounces peeled and deveined large shrimp
½   cup fat-free mayonnaise
⅓   cup fat-free sour cream
1   tablespoon sugar
3   tablespoons lemon juice
1   teaspoon celery seeds
¼   teaspoon salt
¼   teaspoon black pepper
1   (16-ounce) package finely shredded cabbage
¼   cup thinly sliced green bell pepper
¼   cup thinly sliced red onion

Bring water to a boil in a medium saucepan; add shrimp. Cook 3 to 5 minutes or until shrimp are done. Drain well; rinse with cold water.

Combine mayonnaise and next 6 ingredients in a large bowl; stir with a whisk until smooth. Add shrimp, cabbage, green pepper, and onion; toss well. Cover and chill at least 1 hour. **Yield:** 5 servings.

Per Serving:

Calories 115	**Fiber** 2.5g
Fat 0.8g (sat 0.2g)	**Cholesterol** 88mg
Protein 11.9g	**Sodium** 551mg
Carbohydrate 15.2g	**Exchanges:** 1 Starch, 1 Very Lean Meat

For convenience, buy peeled shrimp for this recipe. If you prefer to peel your shrimp, you'll need to buy ¾ pound of unpeeled raw shrimp.

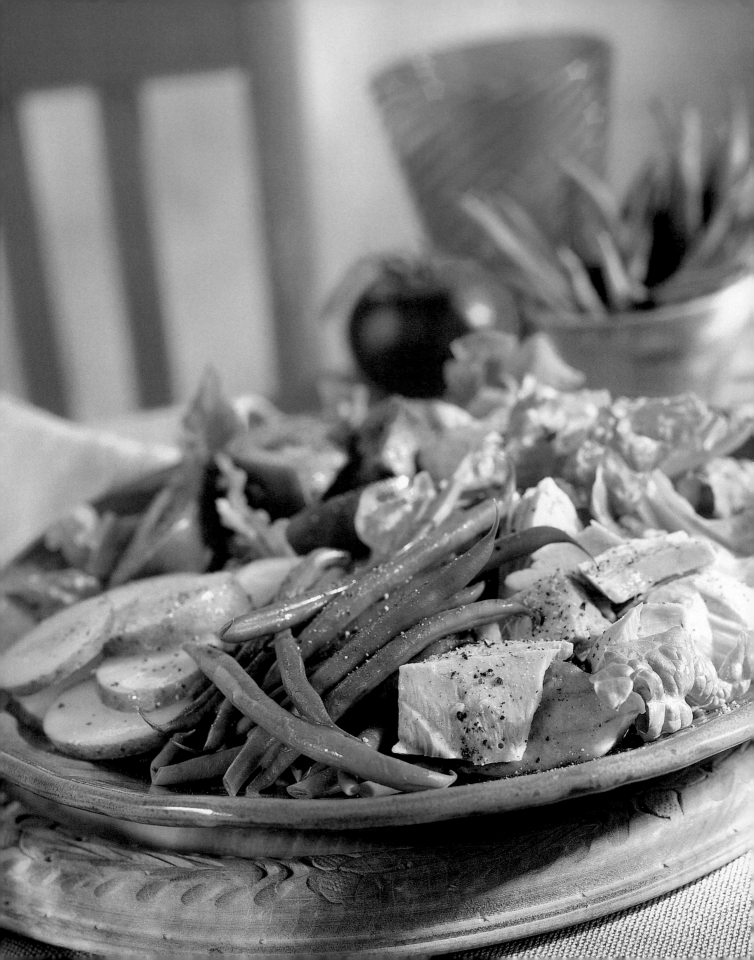

Prep: 17 minutes

Salad Niçoise

¼   pound fresh green beans, trimmed
3   small red potatoes, sliced
1   (8-ounce) tuna steak (¾ inch thick)
⅓   cup white wine vinegar
1½   tablespoons lemon juice
1½   teaspoons Dijon mustard
2   cups torn Bibb lettuce or leaf lettuce
1   tomato, cut into 8 wedges
¼   teaspoon freshly ground black pepper

Arrange green beans and potato on one side of a vegetable steamer over boiling water in a Dutch oven. Place tuna on opposite side of basket. Cover and steam 8 to 10 minutes or until fish flakes easily when tested with a fork. Set tuna aside to cool. Plunge beans and potato into ice water to cool.

Combine vinegar, lemon juice, and mustard in a jar; cover tightly, and shake vigorously.

Place lettuce on a serving platter. Drain potato and beans; arrange over lettuce. Flake tuna, and place on salad; add tomato wedges. Drizzle with vinegar mixture. Sprinkle with freshly ground pepper. **Yield:** 2 servings.

Per Serving:

Calories 279	Fiber 3.8g
Fat 6.2g (sat 1.5g)	Cholesterol 43mg
Protein 30.5g	Sodium 173mg
Carbohydrate 26.5g	Exchanges: 1½ Starch, 1 Vegetable, 4 Very Lean Meat

Prep: 15 minutes

Chinese Chicken Salad

¼   cup sesame seeds, toasted and divided
6   cups shredded cooked chicken breast
1   cup chopped green onions
½   cup fat-free, less-sodium chicken broth
¼   cup fresh lemon juice
1   tablespoon bottled minced ginger
1   tablespoon Chinese mustard
1   teaspoon salt
1   teaspoon "measures-like-sugar" calorie-free sweetener
1   teaspoon ground coriander
1   head green leaf lettuce, shredded

Combine 2 tablespoons sesame seeds and next 9 ingredients in a large saucepan; cook over medium heat until thoroughly heated.

Arrange shredded lettuce on a large platter. Spoon warm chicken mixture over lettuce. Sprinkle 2 tablespoons sesame seeds over chicken mixture. **Yield:** 6 servings (serving size: ¾ cup chicken mixture and about 1 cup lettuce).

Per Serving:

Calories 279	**Fiber** 1.8g
Fat 7.7g (sat 1.8g)	**Cholesterol** 119mg
Protein 45.4g	**Sodium** 357mg
Carbohydrate 5.1g	**Exchanges:** 1 Vegetable, 6 Very Lean Meat

If you don't have leftover chicken to use in this recipe, use deli-roasted chicken breast, or cook about 2 pounds boneless breasts to get 6 cups of shredded chicken.

Prep: 10 minutes   Chill: 2 hours

Cajun Chicken Salad

2½ cups chopped roasted chicken breast
1   cup chopped green bell pepper
¾   cup chopped red or yellow bell pepper
¾   cup chopped red onion
1   cup fat-free mayonnaise
¼   cup country Dijon mustard
1   tablespoon liquid margarine (such as Fleishmann's Light)
1½ teaspoons salt-free Cajun seasoning

Combine all ingredients in a medium bowl; stir well. Cover and chill at least 2 hours. **Yield:** 4 (1-cup) servings.

Per Serving:

Calories 252	**Fiber** 1.7g
Fat 7.4g (sat 1.5g)	**Cholesterol** 74mg
Protein 28.9g	**Sodium** 897mg
Carbohydrate 19.4g	**Exchanges:** 1 Starch, 1 Vegetable, 3 Lean Meat

Look for chopped green, red, and yellow bell peppers on the salad bar at the grocery store.

Prep: 8 minutes   Cook: 4 minutes

Steak Caesar Salad for Two

1   tablespoon no-salt-added lemon pepper seasoning
½   pound boneless beef sirloin steak (¾ inch thick)
Cooking spray
5   cups torn romaine lettuce
¼   cup fat-free seasoned croutons
¼   cup fat-free Caesar-style dressing
6   cherry tomatoes, halved

Rub lemon pepper seasoning on both sides of steak; place steak on rack of a broiler pan coated with cooking spray. Broil 2 to 3 minutes on each side or to desired degree of doneness.

Combine lettuce and remaining 3 ingredients in a large bowl; toss gently. Arrange on 2 salad plates.

Slice steak into thin strips, and arrange over lettuce. **Yield:** *2 servings.*

Per Serving:

Calories 271	**Fiber** 2.0g
Fat 7.1g (sat 2.6g)	**Cholesterol** 80mg
Protein 30.0g	**Sodium** 535mg
Carbohydrate 20.2g	**Exchanges:** ½ Starch, 2 Vegetable, 3 Lean Meat

(Photograph on page 139)

Sides

Herbed Green Beans, page 167

Apple Cider Applesauce • Asparagus with Raspberry Vinaigrette • Pickled Beets
Skillet Cabbage • Herbed Green Beans • Peas and Walnuts
Basil-Lemon Snap Peas • Grilled Bell Peppers
Grilled Summer Squash with Rosemary • Baked Dijon Tomatoes • Waldorf Pilaf
Chilled Red Beans and Rice • Pizzeria Pasta • Pepperoni Pasta Toss

Prep: 10 minutes   Cook: 20 minutes

Apple Cider Applesauce

8   cups sliced peeled cooking apple (about 2½ pounds)
½   cup apple cider or apple juice
¼   cup "measures-like-sugar" calorie-free sweetener
⅛   teaspoon ground nutmeg
¼   teaspoon ground cinnamon

Combine apple and apple cider in a large saucepan. Bring to a boil, stirring frequently; cover, reduce heat, and simmer 20 minutes or until apple is tender, stirring occasionally.

Add sweetener and nutmeg to apple mixture; stir. Cook until sweetener dissolves, stirring constantly. Mash apple mixture slightly with a potato masher until mixture is chunky. Cover and chill thoroughly. Sprinkle evenly with cinnamon before serving. **Yield:** 6 (½-cup) servings.

Per Serving:

Calories 94
Fat 0.5g (sat 0.1g)
Protein 0.2g
Carbohydrate 24.3g
Fiber 2.9g
Cholesterol 0mg
Sodium 1mg
Exchanges: 1½ Fruit

Using a potato masher gets the best chunky texture for this applesauce. If you don't have a potato masher, use a fork.

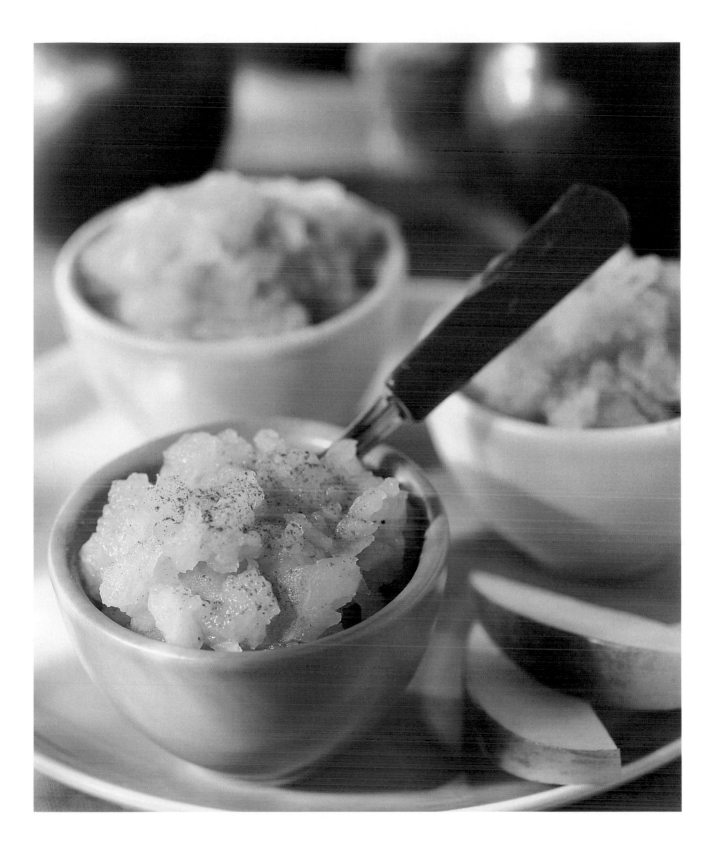

Prep: 5 minutes   Cook: 7 minutes

Asparagus with Raspberry Vinaigrette

1½   pounds asparagus spears
¼   cup raspberry vinegar
1   tablespoon minced shallots
1   tablespoon Dijon mustard
2   teaspoons olive oil
Fresh raspberries (optional)

Snap off tough ends of asparagus. Steam asparagus 7 minutes or until crisp-tender. Drain; transfer to a serving platter.

Combine raspberry vinegar and next 3 ingredients. Pour vinegar mixture over asparagus. Garnish with fresh raspberries, if desired (raspberries not included in analysis). **Yield:** 6 servings.

Per Serving:

Calories 35	**Fiber** 1.6g
Fat 1.8g (sat 0.2g)	**Cholesterol** 0mg
Protein 1.8g	**Sodium** 76mg
Carbohydrate 3.9g	**Exchange:** 1 Vegetable

Asparagus—always a springtime favorite—comes with a bounty of health benefits. It's fat free and low in sodium, and contains fiber, B vitamins, vitamin A, and vitamin C.

Prep: 10 minutes   Cook: 5 minutes

Pickled Beets

2 (14½-ounce) cans sliced beets
½ cup white vinegar
2 tablespoons sugar
4 packets calorie-free sweetener
½ teaspoon salt
¼ teaspoon ground cloves

Drain beets, reserving liquid in a medium saucepan. Discard
½ cup beet liquid. Add beets, vinegar, and remaining ingredients
to the reserved beet liquid in the pan. Bring to a boil; remove
from heat.

Spoon beets into a 1-quart glass jar; pour hot liquid over beets.
Let cool to room temperature. Cover and refrigerate up to 1
month. **Yield:** 7 (½ cup servings).

Per Serving:

Calories 100	**Fiber** 1.3g
Fat 0.1g (sat 0.0g)	**Cholesterol** 0mg
Protein 0.8g	**Sodium** 437mg
Carbohydrate 24.7g	**Exchanges:** 1½ Starch

If you prefer a more subtle clove flavor, reduce
the amount of ground cloves to ⅛ teaspoon.

Skillet Cabbage

2   tablespoons margarine
1   cup chopped onion (about 1)
4   carrots, scraped and cut diagonally into thin slices
6   cups chopped cabbage (about 1 head)
½   cup fat-free, less-sodium chicken broth
½   teaspoon salt
1   teaspoon liquid calorie-free sweetener

Melt margarine in a large nonstick skillet over medium-high heat. Add onion and carrot; sauté 5 minutes or until crisp-tender. Stir in cabbage and remaining ingredients. Bring to a boil; cover, reduce heat, and simmer 11 minutes or until vegetables are tender. **Yield:** 6 (1-cup) servings.

Per Serving:

Calories 85	**Fiber** 3.7g
Fat 4.1g (sat 0.7g)	**Cholesterol** 0mg
Protein 2.3g	**Sodium** 325mg
Carbohydrate 11.4g	**Exchanges:** 2 Vegetable, 1 Fat

Instead of wasting time (and tears) chopping onion, buy a bag of frozen chopped onion to keep on hand.

Prep: 5 minutes   Cook: 10 minutes

Herbed Green Beans

1	pound fresh green beans
2	teaspoons margarine
½	cup sliced green onions
¾	cup presliced mushrooms
2	tablespoons diced pimiento
¼	teaspoon salt
¼	teaspoon pepper
¼	teaspoon dried marjoram
¼	teaspoon dried basil

Trim stem end from beans. Cook beans in boiling water 5 minutes or until crisp-tender. Drain and set aside.

Melt margarine in a large saucepan over medium heat. Add onions and mushrooms; sauté until tender. Add pimiento and remaining 4 ingredients; stir well. Add beans; toss to coat. **Yield:** 4 servings.

Per Serving:

Calories 63	**Fiber** 2.0g
Fat 2.1g (sat 0.3g)	**Cholesterol** 0mg
Protein 3.0g	**Sodium** 179mg
Carbohydrate 10.2g	**Exchanges:** 2 Vegetable

(Photograph on page 161)

Prep: 4 minutes   Cook: 6 minutes

Peas and Walnuts

1   tablespoon light butter
1   large shallot, minced
¼   cup fat-free, less-sodium chicken broth
1   (10-ounce) package frozen green peas, thawed
¼   cup chopped walnuts, toasted
¼   teaspoon salt
¼   teaspoon freshly ground black pepper
¼   teaspoon hot sauce
3   packets calorie-free sweetener

Melt butter in a large skillet over medium-high heat. Add shallots, and sauté 3 minutes. Increase heat to high; add broth and peas. Cook 2 minutes or until liquid evaporates. Stir in walnuts and remaining ingredients. **Yield:** 4 (½-cup) servings.

Per Serving:

Calories 128	**Fiber** 4.0g
Fat 6.7g (sat 1.5g)	**Cholesterol** 5mg
Protein 5.6g	**Sodium** 292mg
Carbohydrate 13.5g	**Exchanges:** 1 Starch, 1 Fat

To toast nuts in the microwave, spread them in a shallow microwave-safe dish; microwave at HIGH 1 to 3 minutes, stopping every 30 seconds to stir.

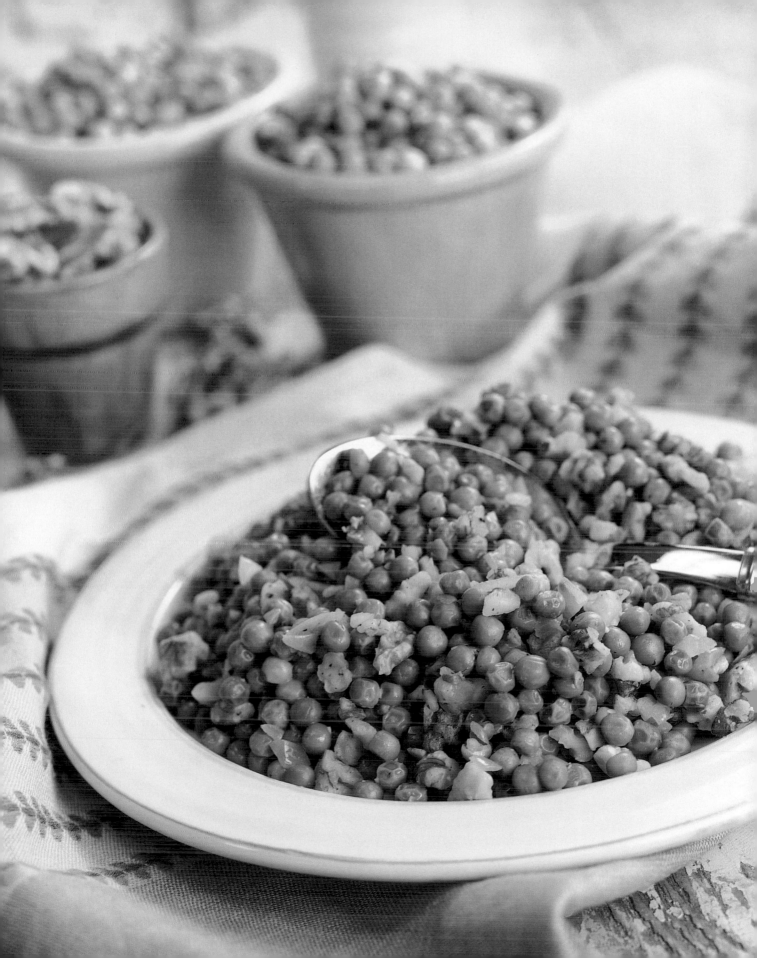

Prep: 10 minutes   Cook: 5 minutes

Basil-Lemon Snap Peas

2	teaspoons olive oil
1	teaspoon bottled minced garlic
1½	pounds sugar snap peas, trimmed
1	cup chopped yellow bell pepper
⅓	cup chopped fresh basil
½	teaspoon sugar
½	teaspoon grated lemon rind
¼	teaspoon salt
¼	teaspoon pepper
2	tablespoons fresh lemon juice

Heat oil in a large nonstick skillet over medium-high heat. Add garlic, and sauté 30 seconds. Add peas and yellow pepper; sauté 2 to 3 minutes or until peas are crisp-tender. Add basil and next 4 ingredients; sauté 30 seconds. Add lemon juice, and sauté 30 seconds. **Yield:** 6 (1-cup) servings.

Per Serving:

Calories 65	**Fiber** 3.0g
Fat 1.8g (sat 0.3g)	**Cholesterol** 0mg
Protein 3.0g	**Sodium** 103mg
Carbohydrate 9.8g	**Exchanges:** 2 Vegetable

One bell pepper—whether it's yellow, red, or green—has more vitamin C than 1 cup of orange juice. Eating foods rich in vitamin C can reduce the risk of heart disease and some cancers.

Prep: 10 minutes   Cook: 30 minutes

Grilled Bell Peppers

3	green bell peppers, coarsely chopped
1	small onion, chopped
1	garlic clove, minced
2	tablespoons grated Parmesan cheese
¼	teaspoon salt
¼	teaspoon dried oregano
¼	teaspoon dried basil
¼	teaspoon dried parsley flakes
¼	teaspoon salt-free herb-and-spice seasoning (such as Mrs. Dash)

Olive oil-flavored cooking spray

Prepare grill.

Combine first 9 ingredients in a bowl.

Coat an 18-inch square of heavy-duty aluminum foil with cooking spray. Spoon vegetable mixture onto foil. Coat vegetables with cooking spray. Close foil around vegetables, sealing tightly.

Place foil packet on grill rack coated with cooking spray; cover and grill 30 minutes, turning packet occasionally. **Yield:** 4 (1-cup) servings.

Per Serving:

Calories 45	Fiber 1.3g
Fat 1.1g (sat 0.6g)	Cholesterol 2mg
Protein 2.3g	Sodium 207mg
Carbohydrate 7.3g	Exchanges: 2 Vegetable

Try this savory side dish as a topping for fajitas.

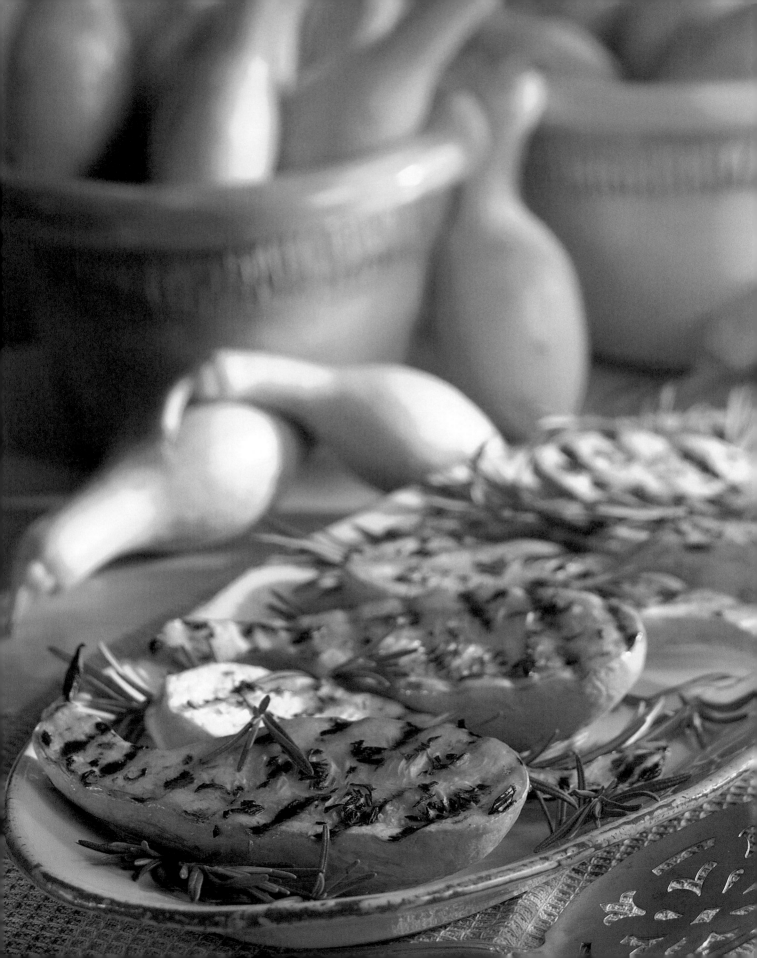

Prep: 5 minutes   Cook: 8 minutes

Grilled Summer Squash with Rosemary

1   pound yellow squash
2   tablespoons balsamic vinegar
1   tablespoon chopped fresh rosemary
1   tablespoon olive oil
¼   teaspoon salt
Olive oil-flavored cooking spray

Prepare grill.

Cut squash in half lengthwise. Combine vinegar and next 3 ingredients in a large bowl. Add squash, and toss to coat.

Place squash on grill rack coated with cooking spray; cover and grill 8 to 10 minutes or until tender, turning and basting with rosemary mixture every 2 minutes. **Yield:** 4 servings.

Per Serving:

Calories 55	**Fiber** 1.5g
Fat 3.7g (sat 0.5g)	**Cholesterol** 0mg
Protein 1.0g	**Sodium** 150mg
Carbohydrate 5.6g	**Exchanges:** 1 Vegetable, ½ Fat

Bright yellow squash is packed with such disease-fighting nutrients as vitamins A and C. And since you eat the skin and the seeds, it's a good source of fiber.

Prep: 7 minutes   Cook: 12 minutes

Baked Dijon Tomatoes

Cooking spray
2   tomatoes, halved crosswise (about 8 ounces each)
2   teaspoons light mayonnaise
2   teaspoons Dijon mustard
Dash of ground red pepper
¼   cup Italian-seasoned breadcrumbs
2   tablespoons chopped fresh parsley
2   tablespoons grated fresh Parmesan cheese

Preheat oven to 400°.

Place tomatoes, cut side up, on a baking sheet coated with cooking spray.

Combine mayonnaise, mustard, and red pepper in a small bowl. Combine breadcrumbs, parsley, and cheese in a second bowl.

Spread about 1 teaspoon mayonnaise mixture on cut sides of each tomato. Top each tomato evenly with breadcrumb mixture. Bake at 400° for 12 to 15 minutes or just until tomato is tender. Remove from oven, and let stand 5 minutes before serving. **Yield:** 4 servings (serving size: 1 tomato half).

Per Serving:

Calories 84	**Fiber** 1.9g
Fat 2.9g (sat 0.8g)	**Cholesterol** 3mg
Protein 3.7g	**Sodium** 263mg
Carbohydrate 12.3g	**Exchanges:** ½ Starch, 1 Vegetable, ½ Fat

Prep: 10 minutes   Cook: 5 minutes

Waldorf Pilaf

1½ cups fat-free, less-sodium chicken broth
½   cup apple juice
½   cup chopped celery
¼   cup chopped onion
1   (6.2-ounce) package fast-cooking recipe long-grain and wild rice
        (such as Uncle Ben's)
¾   cup finely chopped apple
⅓   cup chopped pecans, toasted
3   tablespoons chopped fresh parsley

Combine first 4 ingredients and 1 tablespoon seasoning from rice seasoning packet in a saucepan; discard remaining seasoning.

Bring to a boil; add rice. Cover, reduce heat, and simmer 5 minutes or until liquid is absorbed and rice is tender.

Remove rice mixture from heat; stir in apple, pecans, and parsley. **Yield:** 10 (½-cup) servings.

Per Serving:

Calories 100	**Fiber** 1.1g
Fat 3.0g (sat 0.2g)	**Cholesterol** 2mg
Protein 2.7g	**Sodium** 163mg
Carbohydrate 16.6g	**Exchanges:** 1 Starch, ½ Fat

For a superfast holiday meal, serve this fruited rice with Turkey with Tarragon-Mustard Cream on page 138.

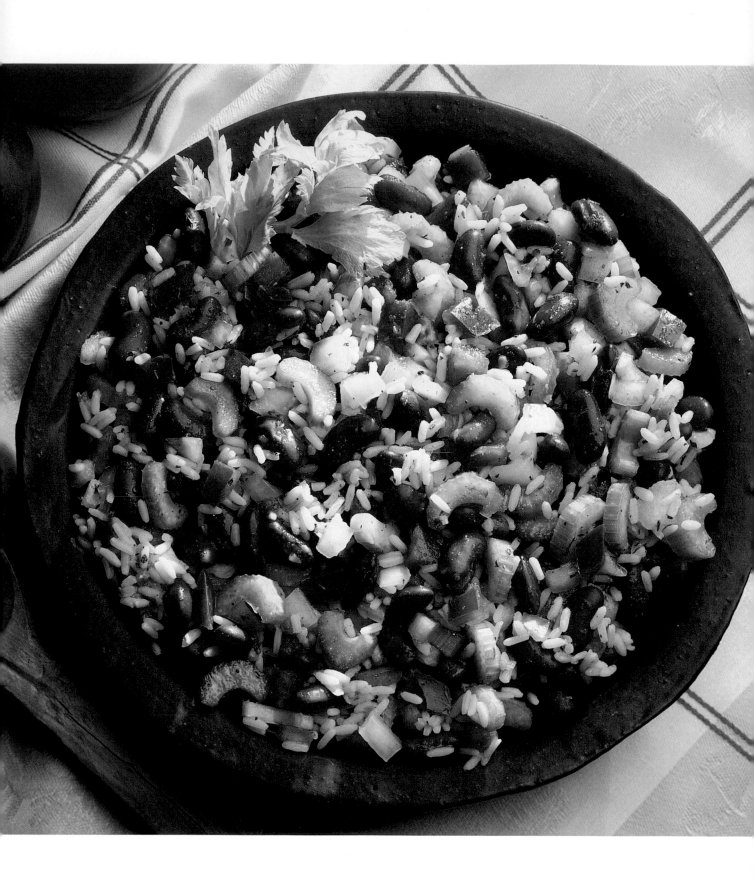

Chilled Red Beans and Rice

¼	cup reduced-fat Italian dressing
3	tablespoons water
2	tablespoons white vinegar
½	teaspoon dried oregano
¼	teaspoon ground red pepper
¼	teaspoon dried thyme
⅛	teaspoon freshly ground black pepper
1	cup cooked long-grain rice, chilled
1	cup sliced celery
¾	cup chopped onion
¾	cup chopped tomato
1	(15-ounce) can red kidney beans, rinsed and drained

Celery leaves (optional)

Combine first 7 ingredients in a jar. Cover tightly, and shake vigorously. Chill.

Combine dressing mixture, rice, and next 4 ingredients in a medium bowl; toss well. Cover and chill. Garnish with celery leaves, if desired. **Yield:** 5 (1-cup) servings.

Per Serving:

Calories 138	**Fiber** 3.3g
Fat 0.7g (sat 0.1g)	**Cholesterol** 0mg
Protein 6.4g	**Sodium** 300mg
Carbohydrate 27.5g	**Exchanges:** 1½ Starch, 1 Vegetable

For rice in a hurry, use 1 regular-size bag of boil-in-bag rice. You'll get 2 cups of cooked rice from 1 bag, so save the rest for another use.

Prep: 10 minutes   Cook: 5 minutes

Pizzeria Pasta

1   (9-ounce) package fresh cheese tortellini
Cooking spray
½   cup chopped green bell pepper
⅓   cup chopped onion
1   (8-ounce) can no-salt-added tomato sauce
¼   cup sliced ripe olives
1   teaspoon dried Italian seasoning
⅛   teaspoon garlic powder

Cook tortellini according to package directions; drain well.

Coat a medium nonstick skillet with cooking spray. Place over medium-high heat until hot. Add pepper and onion; sauté 3 to 4 minutes or until tender.

Stir in tomato sauce and remaining 3 ingredients. Cook over medium-low heat until thoroughly heated, stirring occasionally. Add tomato mixture to tortellini; toss gently. Serve immediately. **Yield:** 6 (½-cup) servings.

Per Serving:

Calories 168	**Fiber** 2.0g
Fat 4.2g (sat 1.2g)	**Cholesterol** 20mg
Protein 7.2g	**Sodium** 246mg
Carbohydrate 24.9g	**Exchanges:** 1 Starch, 2 Vegetable, 1 Fat

Fresh pasta, located in the refrigerated section of the grocery store, cooks in just 5 minutes.

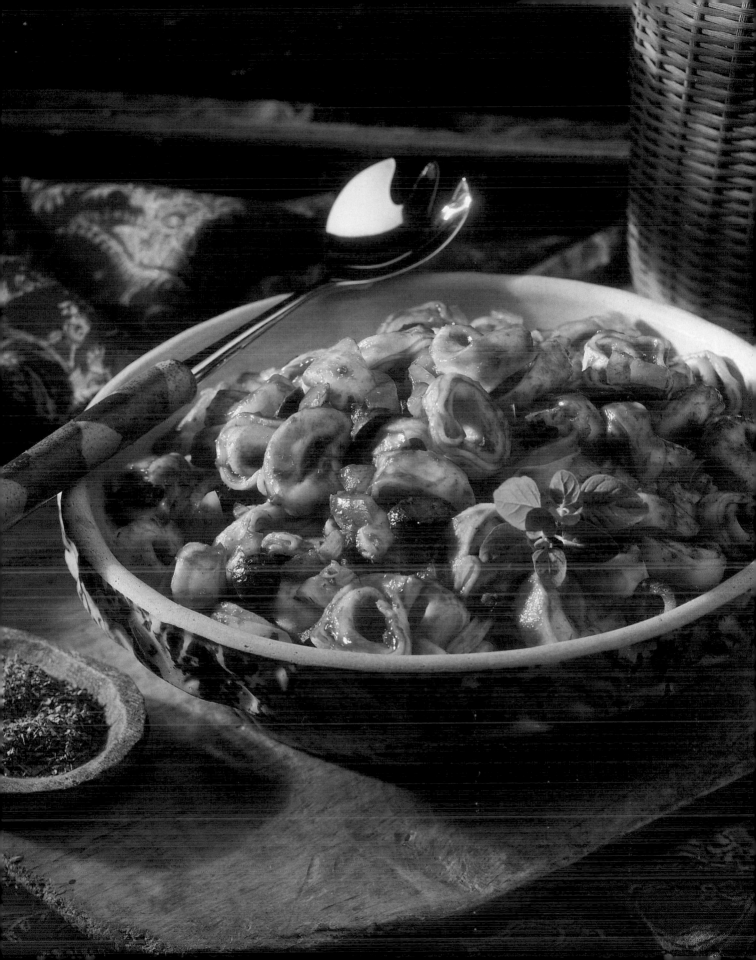

Prep: 1 minute   Cook: 14 minutes

Pepperoni Pasta Toss

8   ounces uncooked spaghetti, broken in half
Cooking spray
1   (8-ounce) package presliced mushrooms
1   (3.5-ounce) package pepperoni, sliced
1   (10-ounce) package fresh spinach, stems removed
⅓   cup fat-free zesty Italian dressing

Cook pasta according to package directions, omitting salt and fat.
Drain well.

Coat a large nonstick skillet with cooking spray; place over
medium-heat until hot. Add mushrooms and pepperoni; sauté until
mushrooms are tender. Add spinach to skillet; cook 2 minutes or
until spinach wilts, stirring often.

Add pasta and dressing to mushroom mixture; toss gently.
Yield: 6 (1-cup) servings.

Per Serving:

Calories 268	**Fiber** 3.3g
Fat 8.2g (sat 2.8g)	**Cholesterol** 14mg
Protein 11.1g	**Sodium** 559mg
Carbohydrate 34.7g	**Exchanges:** 2 Starch, 1 Vegetable, 1½ Fat

Soups & Sandwiches

Round Italian Sandwich, page 199

Chilled Honeydew Soup

5   cups cubed peeled honeydew melon (about ½ melon)
½   cup orange juice
¼   cup sweet white wine
2   tablespoons fresh lime juice
1   tablespoon honey
1   teaspoon grated lime rind

Place melon in a food processor; process until smooth, scraping down sides of bowl occasionally. Transfer melon to a large bowl.

Stir in orange juice and next 3 ingredients. Cover and chill at least 15 minutes. Garnish with grated lime rind. **Yield:** 4 (1-cup) servings.

Per Serving:

Calories 108	**Fiber** 1.2g
Fat 0.2g (sat 0.1g)	**Cholesterol** 0mg
Protein 1.2g	**Sodium** 21mg
Carbohydrate 25.9g	**Exchanges:** 1½ Fruit

To save a little prep time, look for cubed melon in the fresh produce section of the grocery store.

Prep: 5 minutes   Cook: 15 minutes

Corn, Leek, and Potato Chowder

Cooking spray
1   cup sliced leek (about 2 small)
2   cups frozen hash brown potatoes with onions and peppers
         (such as Ore-Ida Potatoes O'Brien), thawed
1   (10-ounce) package frozen whole-kernel corn, thawed
½   teaspoon salt
¼   teaspoon freshly ground black pepper
2½   cups fat-free milk
1   cup (4 ounces) reduced-fat shredded Cheddar cheese

Coat a large saucepan with cooking spray; place over medium-high heat until hot. Add leek, and sauté 2 minutes. Add potatoes and next 3 ingredients; cook 3 minutes, stirring occasionally.

Add milk to potato mixture; bring to a boil. Reduce heat; simmer, uncovered, 8 minutes, stirring often. Ladle chowder into bowls; top each serving with ¼ cup cheese. **Yield:** 4 (1-cup) servings.

Per Serving:

Calories 250	**Fiber** 3.3g
Fat 6.2g (sat 3.4g)	**Cholesterol** 21mg
Protein 17.2g	**Sodium** 603mg
Carbohydrate 34.0g	**Exchanges:** 1½ Starch, 1 Vegetable, 2 Lean Meat

Cook: 18 minutes

Chipotle-Corn Chili

Cooking spray
1   pound coarsely ground round chili meat
¼   teaspoon pepper
1¾ cups frozen whole-kernel corn, thawed
1   (14.5-ounce) can no-salt-added diced tomatoes, undrained
1½ cups bottled thick and chunky chipotle salsa
¾   cup (3 ounces) preshredded reduced-fat Mexican blend
        or Cheddar cheese
2   tablespoons unsalted pumpkinseeds, toasted (optional)

Combine meat and pepper in a small Dutch oven coated with cooking spray. Cook over medium-high heat 10 minutes or until browned, stirring to crumble. Drain, if necessary.

Reduce heat to medium; add corn, and cook, uncovered, 3 minutes, stirring occasionally. Add diced tomatoes and salsa; cook, uncovered, 5 minutes, stirring occasionally. Ladle into each of 4 soup bowls. Top each serving with 3 tablespoons cheese and, if desired, pumpkinseeds. **Yield:** 4 (1¼-cup) servings.

Per Serving:

Calories 334	**Fiber** 2.9g
Fat 14.2g (sat 6.4g)	**Cholesterol** 49mg
Protein 31.6g	**Sodium** 942mg
Carbohydrate 22.5g	**Exchanges:** 1½ Starch, 4 Lean Meat

Look for pumpkinseeds in health food stores, Mexican markets, or supermarkets. You can buy them in a variety of forms: salted, unsalted, roasted, raw, and with or without nuts.

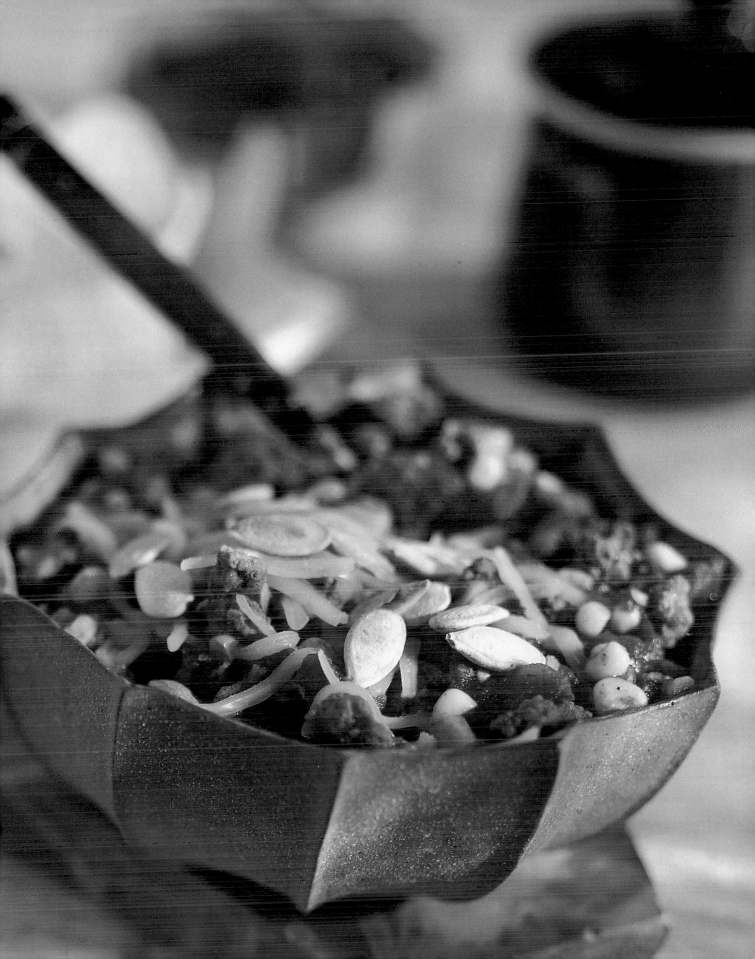

Prep: 3 minutes   Cook: 10 minutes

Beefy Minestrone Soup

²⁄₃ cup uncooked ditalini (very short tube-shaped macaroni)
2   (14.25-ounce) cans fat-free, less-sodium beef broth
1   (14.5-ounce) can no-salt-added stewed tomatoes, undrained
1   large zucchini
1   (15.5-ounce) can cannellini beans or other white beans, rinsed
         and drained
2   teaspoons dried Italian seasoning
8   ounces deli rare roast beef, sliced ¼-inch-thick and diced

Combine first 3 ingredients in a large saucepan; cover and bring
to a boil over high heat.

Cut zucchini in half lengthwise, and slice. Add zucchini, beans,
and Italian seasoning to pasta; cover, reduce heat, and simmer
6 minutes. Add beef, and cook 4 minutes or until pasta is tender.
Yield: 6 (1½-cup) servings.

Per Serving:

Calories 157	**Fiber** 4.4g
Fat 1.8g (sat 0.7g)	**Cholesterol** 20mg
Protein 13.5g	**Sodium** 303mg
Carbohydrate 20.7g	**Exchanges:** 1 Starch, 1 Vegetable, 1 Very Lean Meat

Prep: 6 minutes   Cook: 8 minutes

Mexican Chicken Soup

5	cups fat-free, less-sodium chicken broth
1½	cups bottled thick and chunky salsa
1	(9-ounce) package frozen diced cooked chicken breast, thawed
1	cup rinsed and drained no-salt-added canned black beans
1	cup uncooked instant rice
¼	cup chopped fresh cilantro
2	tablespoons fresh lime juice
¾	cup coarsely crushed low-fat baked tortilla chips

Bring broth and salsa to a boil in a large, heavy saucepan over high heat. Add chicken, beans, and rice; cover, reduce heat to low, and cook 5 minutes or until rice is tender. Remove from heat; stir in cilantro and lime juice.

Spoon soup evenly into bowls. Sprinkle each serving with 2 tablespoons chips. **Yield:** 6 servings (serving size: about 2 cups).

Per Serving:

Calories 245	**Fiber** 2.5g
Fat 3.6g (sat 0.9g)	**Cholesterol** 49mg
Protein 25.6g	**Sodium** 816mg
Carbohydrate 26.5g	**Exchanges:** 1½ Starch, 3 Very Lean Meat

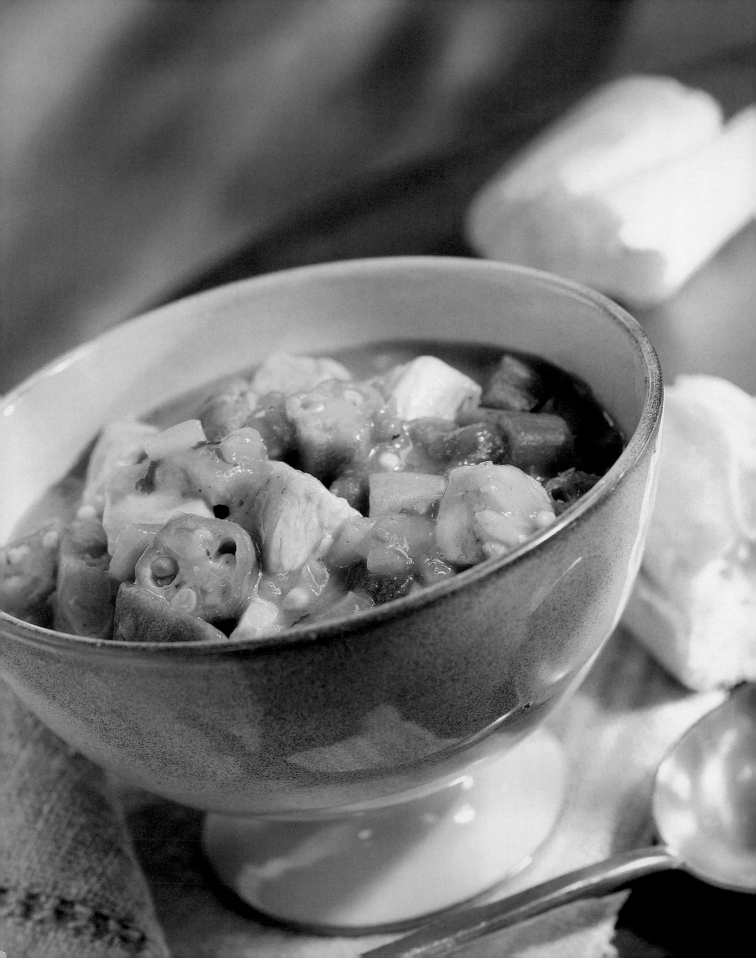

Prep: 2 minutes   Cook: 14 minutes

Quick Chicken Gumbo

1   teaspoon olive oil
1   (10-ounce) package frozen chopped onion, celery, and pepper
       blend
2   tablespoons all-purpose flour
1   cup fat-free, less-sodium chicken broth
¼   teaspoon hot sauce
1   (14.5-ounce) can Cajun-style stewed tomatoes with pepper, garlic,
       and Cajun spices, undrained
1   (10-ounce) package frozen cut okra
1½   cups frozen diced cooked chicken breast

Heat olive oil in a large nonstick skillet over medium-high heat. Add frozen vegetable blend, and sauté 3 minutes.

Add flour, stirring well. Add chicken broth, hot sauce, and tomatoes; cook 3 minutes or until mixture is slightly thickened. Add okra and chicken; cover and cook 8 minutes or until okra is tender.
Yield: 5 (1-cup) servings.

Per Serving:

Calories 164	**Fiber** 2.0g
Fat 3.1g (sat 0.6g)	**Cholesterol** 33mg
Protein 16.8g	**Sodium** 462mg
Carbohydrate 16.8g	**Exchanges:** 3 Vegetable, 2 Very Lean Meat

Oyster Po'Boy

⅓   cup white cornmeal
⅓   cup dry breadcrumbs
1½   teaspoons salt-free Cajun seasoning
2   (8-ounce) containers standard oysters, well drained
Cooking spray
1   tablespoon vegetable oil, divided
1   (8-ounce) unsliced loaf French bread
¼   cup light mayonnaise
3   tablespoons Creole mustard
1½   cups thinly sliced romaine lettuce
1   tomato, thinly sliced

Combine first 3 ingredients in a bowl; stir well. Dredge oysters in cornmeal mixture.

Heat 1½ teaspoons oil in a large nonstick skillet coated with cooking spray over medium heat. Add half of oysters, and cook 3 minutes on each side or until oysters are done and breading is golden. Repeat with 1½ teaspoons oil and remaining oysters.

Cut bread in half horizontally, and spread mayonnaise and mustard evenly over cut sides of bread. Arrange lettuce and tomato slices over bottom half of loaf. Top with cooked oysters and top half of loaf. Cut loaf into 4 pieces. Serve immediately. **Yield:** 4 servings.

Per Serving:

Calories 351	**Fiber** 3.2g
Fat 9.3g (sat 1.7g)	**Cholesterol** 52mg
Protein 14.3g	**Sodium** 845mg
Carbohydrate 50.7g	**Exchanges:** 3 Starch, 1 Vegetable, ½ Lean Meat, 1 Fat

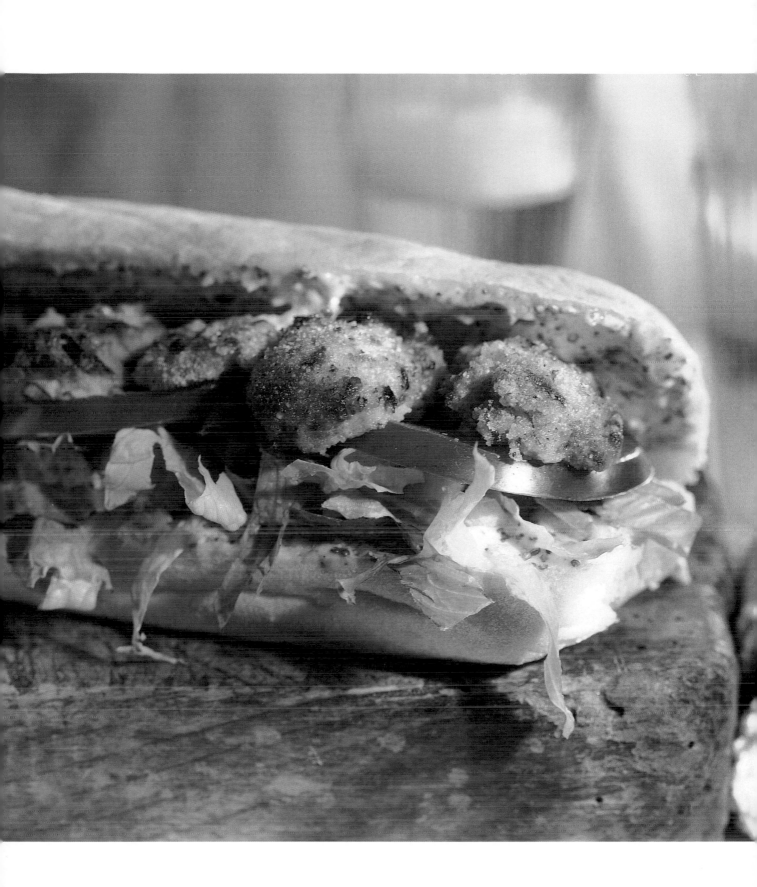

*super*Quick

Prep: 10 minutes   Cook: 6 minutes

Grilled Vegetable Pita Sandwiches

1   tablespoon olive oil
1   teaspoon dried Italian seasoning
1   teaspoon dried parsley flakes
¼   teaspoon salt
¼   teaspoon pepper
1   zucchini, cut lengthwise into ¼-inch-thick slices
1   eggplant, cut lengthwise into ¼-inch-thick slices
1   yellow squash, cut lengthwise into ¼-inch-thick slices
1   small purple onion, cut into ¼-inch-thick slices
Cooking spray
1   tomato, thinly sliced
4   (6-inch) pitas, cut in half
1   cup broccoli or alfalfa sprouts
½   cup (2 ounces) reduced-fat shredded Monterey Jack cheese
½   cup reduced-fat ranch dressing

Combine first 5 ingredients in a small bowl. Brush zucchini,
eggplant, yellow squash, and onion with oil mixture.

Prepare grill. Place vegetables on grill rack coated with cooking
spray; cover and grill 6 minutes or until tender, turning once.

Layer grilled vegetables and tomato evenly in pita halves. Fill each
pita half with 2 tablespoons sprouts; top with 1 tablespoon each
of cheese and dressing. **Yield:** 8 servings (serving size: 1 filled
pita half).

Per Serving:

Calories 215	Fiber 3.6g
Fat 8.4g (sat 2.4g)	Cholesterol 14mg
Protein 9.1g	Sodium 503mg
Carbohydrate 27.1g	Exchanges: 2 Starch, ½ Medium-Fat Meat, 1 Fat

Prep: 3 minutes   Cook: 25 minutes

Barbecue Beef Sandwiches

1   pound ground round
½   cup chopped onion
1   (8-ounce) can tomato sauce
¼   cup white vinegar
1   teaspoon prepared mustard
1   packet calorie-free sweetener
5   (1½-ounce) hamburger buns

Cook meat and onion in a nonstick skillet over medium-high heat until meat is browned and onion is tender, stirring to crumble meat.

Stir in tomato sauce and next 3 ingredients. Cover, reduce heat, and simmer 20 minutes, stirring occasionally. Spoon meat mixture evenly onto hamburger buns. **Yield:** 5 servings.

Per Serving:

Calories 294
Fat 10.4g (sat 3.8g)
Protein 23.0g
Carbohydrate 25.9g

Fiber 2.0g
Cholesterol 33mg
Sodium 579mg
Exchanges: 1½ Starch, 1 Vegetable, 2 Medium-Fat Meat

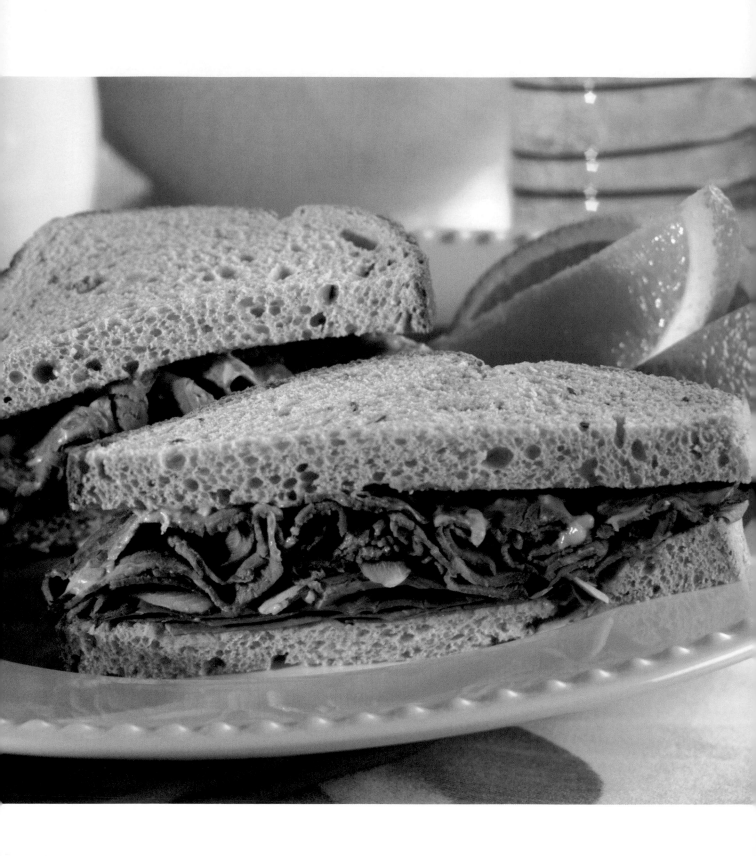

Prep: 9 minutes   Chill: 1 hour

Oriental Beef on Rye

2   tablespoons fat-free mayonnaise
2   tablespoons low-sodium teriyaki sauce
2   teaspoons bottled minced ginger
1   garlic clove, minced
6   (1-ounce) slices rye bread
½   cup spinach leaves
2   tablespoons sliced almonds, toasted
9   ounces thinly sliced 98% fat-free deli roast beef

Combine first 4 ingredients, mixing well. Spread 1 teaspoon mayonnaise mixture on each of 3 bread slices. Top each with spinach leaves and almonds. Drizzle each sandwich with 2 teaspoons mayonnaise mixture. Arrange roast beef evenly on sandwiches. Drizzle each sandwich with 1 teaspoon remaining mayonnaise mixture; top with remaining bread slices. Wrap each sandwich in plastic wrap, and chill at least 1 hour. **Yield:** 3 servings.

Per Serving:

Calories 225	**Fiber** 3.4g
Fat 3.8g (sat 0.1g)	**Cholesterol** 23mg
Protein 10.9g	**Sodium** 979mg
Carbohydrate 40.4g	**Exchanges:** 2½ Starch, 1 Lean Meat

Ask for thin slices of 98% fat-free deli roast beef at the deli counter in your supermarket.

Prep: 12 minutes

Dilled Chicken Salad Sandwiches

½   cup plain fat-free yogurt
2   cups chopped cooked chicken
¼   cup chopped celery
¼   cup chopped green onions
1   tablespoon honey mustard
¼   teaspoon dried dill
¼   teaspoon pepper
4   leaf lettuce leaves
8   (1-ounce) slices whole wheat bread, lightly toasted
4   (¼-inch-thick) slices large tomato

Spoon yogurt onto several layers of heavy-duty paper towels; spread to ½-inch thickness. Cover with additional paper towels; let stand 5 minutes. Scrape into a medium bowl, using a rubber spatula.

Add chicken and next 5 ingredients to yogurt; stir well. Place lettuce leaves over 4 bread slices; top with chicken mixture, tomato slices, and remaining bread slices. **Yield:** 4 servings.

Per Serving:

Calories 323	**Fiber** 3.5g
Fat 7.8g (sat 2.0g)	**Cholesterol** 64mg
Protein 28.1g	**Sodium** 410mg
Carbohydrate 34.5g	**Exchanges:** 2 Starch, 3 Lean Meat

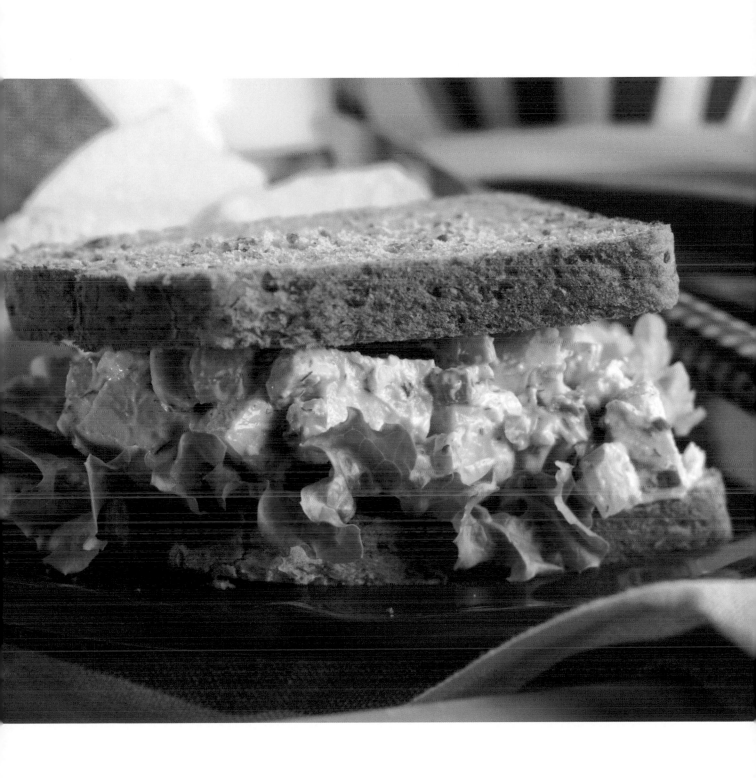

superQuick

Prep: 5 minutes   Cook: 10 minutes

Hickory-Grilled Chicken Sandwiches

4   (4-ounce) skinless, boneless chicken breast halves
4   (¼-inch-thick) slices red onion
⅓   cup hickory-flavored barbecue sauce
Cooking spray
4   canned pineapple slices
4   reduced-calorie hamburger buns

Prepare grill.

Brush chicken and onion with barbecue sauce. Place chicken, onion, and pineapple on grill rack coated with cooking spray; cover and grill 5 minutes on each side or until chicken is done, removing onion and pineapple when tender.

Place each chicken breast on a bottom half of bun; top with onion, pineapple, and top half of bun. **Yield:** 4 servings.

Per Serving:

Calories 276
Fat 4.4g (sat 1.0g)
Protein 30.2g
Carbohydrate 30.3g

Fiber 3.8g
Cholesterol 70mg
Sodium 421mg
Exchanges: 1½ Starch, ½ Fruit, 3 Very Lean Meat

Prep: 12 minutes   Chill: 1 hour

Round Italian Sandwich

1   (6½-inch) round loaf sourdough bread (about 8 ounces)
2   (1-ounce) slices provolone cheese, halved
2   slices turkey salami, halved
1   slice turkey ham, halved
2   small tomatoes, thinly sliced
2   cups torn spinach
2   tablespoons balsamic vinegar
2   tablespoons grated Parmesan cheese
½   teaspoon freshly ground black pepper

Slice bread horizontally into 3 equal layers, using an electric or serrated knife. Layer half each of provolone cheese, salami, ham, tomato, and spinach on bottom slice of bread. Sprinkle spinach with half each of balsamic vinegar, Parmesan cheese, and pepper; top with second bread slice. Repeat procedure with remaining provolone cheese, salami, ham, tomato, and spinach. Sprinkle spinach with remaining balsamic vinegar, Parmesan cheese, and pepper; top with remaining bread slice.

Wrap sandwich tightly in plastic wrap, and chill at least 1 hour. To serve, slice sandwich into 4 wedges. **Yield:** 4 servings.

Per Serving:

Calories 256	**Fiber** 2.6g
Fat 7.5g (sat 3.4g)	**Cholesterol** 24mg
Protein 13.7g	**Sodium** 698mg
Carbohydrate 34.5g	**Exchanges:** 2 Starch, 1 Vegetable, 1 Medium-Fat Meat

(Photograph on page 181)

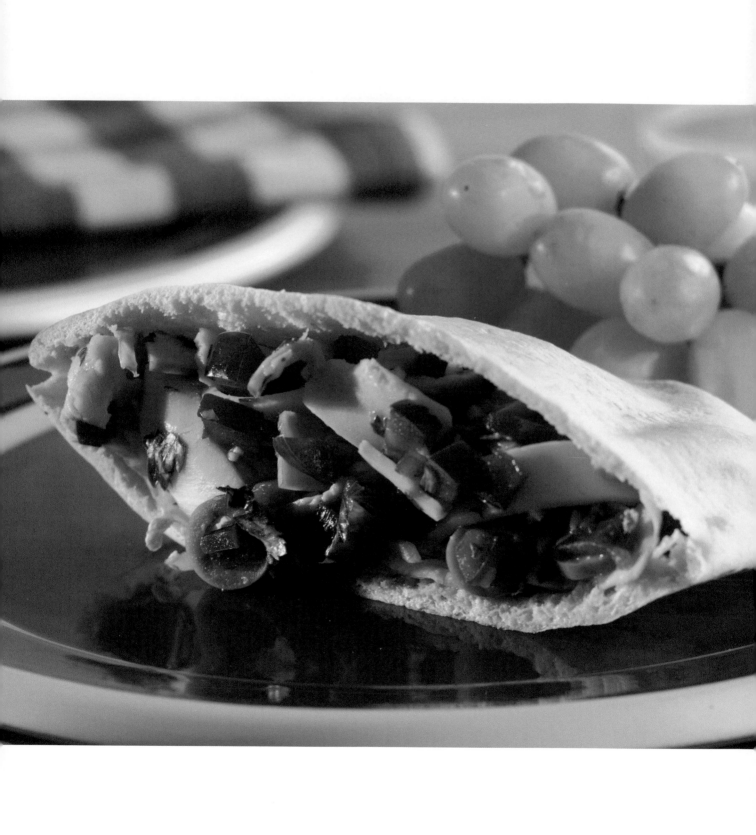

make *Ahead*

Prep: 9 minutes   Chill: 1 hour

Turkey Muffuletta Pitas

3	ounces thinly sliced smoked turkey, cut into strips
2	ounces thinly sliced provolone cheese, cut into strips
1½	cups finely chopped red bell pepper
⅓	cup sliced pimiento-stuffed olives
¼	cup chopped fresh parsley
2	tablespoons fat-free Italian dressing
2	tablespoons red wine vinegar
3	small garlic cloves, minced
1	cup shredded lettuce
2	(6-inch) pitas, cut in half

Combine first 8 ingredients in a medium bowl; toss well. Cover and chill at least 1 hour.

Spoon lettuce evenly into pita halves. Spoon turkey mixture evenly on top of lettuce. **Yield:** 4 servings.

Per Serving:

Calories 189	**Fiber** 4.4g
Fat 5.8g (sat 2.8g)	**Cholesterol** 22mg
Protein 11.1g	**Sodium** 533mg
Carbohydrate 22.1g	**Exchanges:** 1 Starch, 1 Vegetable, 1 Medium-Fat Meat

Mix up the tangy filling for this pocket sandwich in advance. When you're ready to eat, just spoon in the filling, and you've got a sandwich in seconds!

Recipe Index

See page 206 for list of SuperQuick and
Make-Ahead Recipes.

super*Quick* Recipes (20 minutes or less)

make *Ahead* Recipes

Nutrition Notes

Quick & Easy Diabetic Recipes gives you the nutrition facts you want to know. We provide the following information with every recipe.

values are for one serving of the recipe

Per Serving:

Calories 299

Fat 2.0g (sat 0.4g)

Protein 22.8g

total carbohydrate in one serving

Carbohydrate 29.1g

Fiber 2.0g — grams are abbreviated "g"

Cholesterol 47 mg — milligrams are abbreviated "mg"

Sodium 644mg

Exchanges: 2 Starch, 2 Medium-Fat Meat — exchange values are for one serving

Nutritional Analyses

The nutritional values used in our calculations either come from a nutrient analysis computer program or are provided by food manufacturers. The values are based on the following assumptions:

- When we give a range for an ingredient, we calculate using the lesser amount.

- Only the amount of marinade absorbed is calculated.

- Garnishes and optional ingredients are not included in the analysis.

Diabetic Exchanges

Exchange values for all recipes are provided for people who use them for meal planning. The exchange values in this book are based on the *Exchange Lists for Meal Planning* developed by the American Diabetes Association and The American Dietetic Association.

Carbohydrate

If you count carbohydrate, look for the value in the nutrient analysis. The new American Diabetes Association guidelines loosen the restriction on sugar and encourage you to look at the total grams of carbohydrate in a serving. We have used small amounts of sugar in some recipes. We have also used a variety of sugar substitutes when the use of a substitute yields a quality product (see the Sugar Substitute Guide on page 18).

Sodium

Current dietary recommendations advise a daily sodium intake of 2,400 milligrams. We have limited the sodium in these recipes by using reduced-sodium products whenever possible.

If you must restrict sodium in your diet, please note the sodium value per serving and see if you should further modify the recipe.

metric equivalents

The recipes that appear in this cookbook use the standard United States method for measuring liquid and dry or solid ingredients (teaspoons, tablespoons, and cups). The information in the following charts is provided to help cooks outside the U.S. successfully use these recipes. All equivalents are approximate.

Equivalents for Different Types of Ingredients

A standard cup measure of a dry or solid ingredient will vary in weight depending on the type of ingredient. A standard cup of liquid is the same volume for any type of liquid. Use the following chart when converting standard cup measures to grams (weight) or milliliters (volume).

Standard Cup	Fine Powder (ex. flour)	Grain (ex. rice)	Granular (ex. sugar)	Liquid Solids (ex. butter)	Liquid (ex. milk)
1	140 g	150 g	190 g	200 g	240 ml
¾	105 g	113 g	143 g	150 g	180 ml
⅔	93 g	100 g	125 g	133 g	160 ml
½	70 g	75 g	95 g	100 g	120 ml
⅓	47 g	50 g	63 g	67 g	80 ml
¼	35 g	38 g	48 g	50 g	60 ml
⅛	18 g	19 g	24 g	25 g	30 ml

Liquid Ingredients by Volume

¼ tsp					1 ml
½ tsp					2 ml
1 tsp					5 ml
3 tsp	= 1 tbls		= ½ fl oz	=	15 ml
	2 tbls	= ⅛ cup	= 1 fl oz	=	30 ml
	4 tbls	= ¼ cup	= 2 fl oz	=	60 ml
	5⅓ tbls	= ⅓ cup	= 3 fl oz	=	80 ml
	8 tbls	= ½ cup	= 4 fl oz	=	120 ml
	10⅔ tbls	= ⅔ cup	= 5 fl oz	=	160 ml
	12 tbls	= ¾ cup	= 6 fl oz	=	180 ml
	16 tbls	= 1 cup	= 8 fl oz	=	240 ml
1 pt	= 2 cups	= 16 fl oz	=	480 ml	
1 qt	= 4 cups	= 32 fl oz	=	960 ml	
		33 fl oz	= 1000 ml	= 1 liter	

Dry Ingredients by Weight

(To convert ounces to grams, multiply the number of ounces by 30.)

1 oz	=	¹⁄₁₆ lb	=	30 g
4 oz	=	¼ lb	=	120 g
8 oz	=	½ lb	=	240 g
12 oz	=	¾ lb	=	360 g
16 oz	=	1 lb	=	480 g

Length

(To convert inches to centimeters, multiply the number of inches by 2.5.)

1 in =			2.5 cm	
6 in =	½ ft	=	15 cm	
12 in =	1 ft	=	30 cm	
36 in =	3 ft = 1 yd	=	90 cm	
40 in =			100 cm	= 1 m

Cooking/Oven Temperatures

	Fahrenheit	Celsius	Gas Mark
Freeze Water	32° F	0° C	
Room Temperature	68° F	20° C	
Boil Water	212° F	100° C	
Bake	325° F	160° C	3
	350° F	180° C	4
	375° F	190° C	5
	400° F	200° C	6
	425° F	220° C	7
	450° F	230° C	8
Broil			Grill